DOG DOCTOR

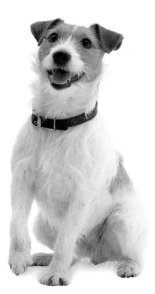

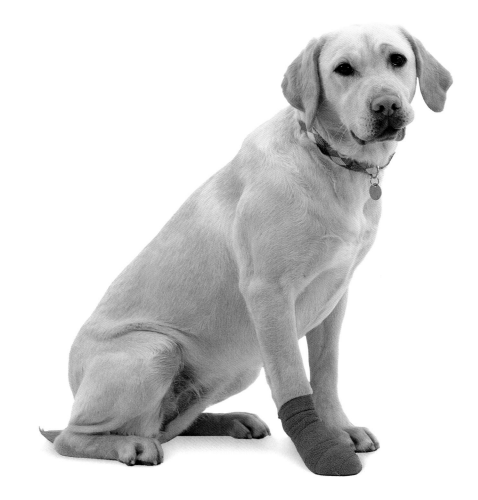

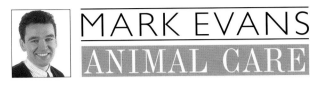

MARK EVANS
ANIMAL CARE

DOG DOCTOR

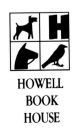

HOWELL
BOOK
HOUSE

To Anna and Tom

First published in Great Britain in 1996 by Mitchell Beazley,
an imprint of Reed Consumer Books Limited,
Michelin House, 81 Fulham Road, London SW3 6RB and
Auckland, Melbourne, Singapore and Toronto

Howell Book House
A Simon & Schuster Macmillan Company
1633 Broadway
New York, NY 10019

MACMILLAN is a registered trademark of Macmillan, Inc.

ISBN 0-87605-678-8

Library of Congress Cataloging-in-Publication
data available upon request

Printed in China

10 9 8 7 6 5 4 3 2 1

Contents

Introduction

When your dog is unwell, your concern for his welfare may be no less than it would be if a human member of your family were ill or injured. In fact, in my experience, owners are often more worried when their dogs are unwell than they would be if they were ill themselves, and there is no doubt in my mind that their concerns are often fuelled by feelings of helplessness and lack of knowledge.

The aim of this book is to encourage you to take a more pro-active role in your dog's medical care. The better informed you are about common dog ailments – including their major causes and symptoms, and the most up-to-date veterinary services and procedures available to diagnose, treat and prevent them – the better able you will be to make the right healthcare choices on behalf of your dog.

You will also be a more valuable member of your dog's medical team when he is unwell and, as a result, you are sure to feel less frustrated and much more helpful at the times when he needs you most.

Your dog's health

Despite what many people may think, dogs are as complex as humans in the way their bodies are built and in the way they work. Although humans and dogs may have very different mental abilities, we and they are both mammals and, from an anatomical and purely functional point of view, we have much in common with our four-legged friends. Just like us, dogs are vulnerable to injuries of all kinds, and to a very large number of specific diseases. When they are unwell, they suffer as we do.

Caring for your dog is a team responsibility and, together with the staff at your vet centre, you are an essential part of that team. However, despite your best efforts to keep him healthy, it is likely that sooner or later your dog will suffer from an accidental injury or illness of some kind. After all, it is a rare individual indeed – either human or canine – who manages to go through a lifetime without medical problems.

When your dog is off-colour he will rely on you to identify that there is something wrong with him, and to take prompt and appropriate action. Although a vet will be the only person suitably qualified to diagnose the cause and full extent of your dog's symptoms, and to instigate treatment, you will be the person who is able to give your vet essential information concerning the history and symptoms of your dog's illness or injury. For instance, if your dog suffers from a severe bout of vomiting, it will help your vet to diagnose the cause if you are able to tell him or her when your dog has vomited, and the nature of what he has produced.

It is very likely that you will also play a crucial role in nursing your dog through recovery from illness, and in monitoring his progress to report back to your vet.

Seeking veterinary help

Make no mistake, this book is certainly not intended to encourage you to avoid seeking advice and practical assistance from your vet centre when your dog is injured or ill. There is nothing more dangerous to a dog's welfare than an owner who, armed with only half the facts, refuses to recognize the limitations of his or her knowledge about dog health and fails to seek professional veterinary care for his or her pet when required. For your dog's sake, you must be prepared to talk to someone at your vet centre promptly whenever you are at all concerned about his health or welfare, no matter how trivial you think the problem may be.

Our knowledge and understanding of dogs – and therefore our ability to look after them in the best way possible – will only improve through continued research into their anatomy, behaviour and the ways in which their bodies work.

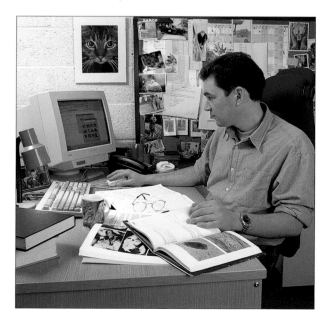

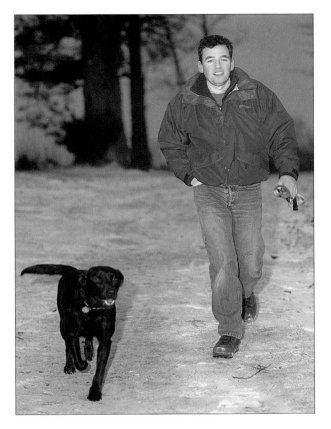

The author walking near his home with his three-year-old labrador retriever, Jessie.

Using this book

The first section of the book explains the importance of regularly monitoring your dog's health in order to identify at an early stage the signs and symptoms of ill-health. When your dog is off-colour, taking action quickly will prevent him from suffering unnecessarily, and could even save his life. A quick reference table of some of the possible causes of a number of the most common symptoms suffered by ill or injured dogs is provided to help you to organize your thoughts.

It may surprise you to discover that, in the UK at least, no-one seems to know for certain what the most common medical conditions suffered by dogs actually are. As a result, the conditions included in this book are based on the combined opinions of 180 veterinary surgeons employed by the People's Dispensary for Sick Animals (PDSA).

When your dog is ill, you may find it difficult to consider at the time, or to remember in detail later on, all the specific information and advice dispensed by your vet or a veterinary nurse during a consultation or over the telephone. In my experience, even the most level-headed owners show an understandable lack of mental clarity when their thoughts are clouded by overriding concerns for their dogs' welfare.

The information provided in relation to each of the conditions included in the second section of the book is intended to be considered in conjunction with specific advice offered by the staff at your vet centre. This information will help you to understand not only the condition from which your dog is suffering, but also the diagnostic procedures and treatments to which he may be subjected, and the kind of nursing care that he is likely to need from you at home.

Choosing the right vet centre for your dog is an essential first step in providing him with the very best of healthcare. As you might expect, vet centres vary considerably, not only in the services that they offer but also in how they deliver them. It is up to you to undertake the proper research to find a vet centre in your area that you believe will be well-suited both to you and to your dog. You will find information on choosing and using veterinary services in section three.

The section on special care covers the most common practical nursing procedures that may be involved in caring at home for the medical needs of ill dogs, from administering medicines to changing simple dressings.

As some of the most common conditions suffered by dogs are to a large degree preventable, the special-care section also brings into focus the importance of preventive healthcare. With the guidance of the staff at your vet centre, you should put together a preventive-healthcare plan for your dog that is tailored to his own particular needs and lifestyle. Your vet centre should also be able to provide you with a range of items such as parasite-control and dental-care products, and even foods formulated to help in treating certain conditions.

If your dog – or someone else's dog – is involved in an accident or other emergency and you are the first person on the scene, being able to carry out basic first aid could save the dog's life. The first-aid section at the end of the book is a quick, practical reference guide to what to do in some of the most common emergency situations in which dogs may be involved, such as road-traffic accidents. You should familiarize yourself with the information that this section contains now, before you even put this book down: you never know when you may suddenly need to refer to it.

Signs and symptoms

Recognizing early symptoms of illness or injury in your dog is vital. By carrying out routine health-checks, you will become familiar with how he looks, feels and smells, so that you will spot any unusual signs as soon as they appear. You can then take prompt action to ensure that your dog does not suffer unnecessarily.

Identifying symptoms

As your dog's owner you have two important roles. The first is to keep him healthy by feeding him a good diet, giving him plenty of exercise and mental stimulation, grooming him regularly, treating him for common parasites and keeping him up to date with vaccinations. The second is to monitor his behaviour and his inputs and outputs, and to carry out regular anatomical checks to identify the first signs of illness.

BEHAVIOUR

A change in your dog's behaviour may be significant. If he grooms himself more than usual, there could be something wrong with his skin or coat; if he will not jump into the car as he normally does, it could be that something hurts; if he is suddenly dull and depressed, he is very likely to be ill. Not all symptoms are this obvious, but you should never ignore a behavioural change in your dog, no matter how trivial it may seem.

INPUTS AND OUTPUTS

Changes in your dog's normal eating, drinking and toileting habits may occur as a result of a number of medical and psychological conditions.

CONTACTING YOUR VET CENTRE

Do not hesitate to contact your vet centre if you are worried about your dog. Your vet or a veterinary nurse will give you advice over the telephone and, if you are worrying needlessly, will put your mind at rest. If your concerns are valid, he or she will tell you what to do.

Never be embarrassed to ask questions. No-one is born with an in-built knowledge of dog anatomy and healthcare, and, if you don't ask, you won't learn.

Food

Lack of appetite, or complete anorexia (refusal to eat), is an obvious symptom of illness, but so too is the development of fussy or ravenous feeding behaviour.

Water

If your dog is drinking much more water than normal, measure his intake over 24 hours (see page 110).

It is considered to be abnormal for a dog to drink more than 100 ml (3 fl oz) of water per day for each kilogramme (2 lb 3 oz) of his body weight.

Urine and faeces

Get to know your dog's toileting habits and the nature of what he normally produces. Look out for changes in the colour or consistency of his faeces. If you notice anything unusual in his urine, ask at your vet centre for a special collecting device (see page 66), and obtain a sample for your vet or a veterinary nurse to analyse.

ANATOMY

Aim to carry out a basic health-check on your dog once a week. The order in which you undertake each check does not matter, as long as you are methodical. In time, you will find that you are doing some of the examinations almost subconsciously while you are stroking or grooming your dog.

Carry out health-checks in good light, preferably with your dog on a suitable table. Use not only your eyes, but also your fingers and nose to gain information about your dog's condition. For instance, the first sign of an ear infection could be a noticeable odour at one of his ear holes, while tiny scabs that develop in some skin disorders can be easier to feel than they are to see.

Simple checks

Watch your dog breathing: the respiratory rate of a healthy dog is usually between 10 and 30 breaths per minute at rest. Run your hands firmly over your dog's whole body, including up his legs, under his chest and stomach and along his tail. As you move your fingers along his chest just behind his elbows you may feel his heartbeat. If so, count the beats: most healthy dogs have a heart-rate of 70–140 beats per minute at rest.

Be sensitive to your dog's reactions as you examine him: a quick turn of his head may be the only sign that he will give of a painful spot.

Check your dog's skin and coat: any crusts and scabs may feel as though sugar has been sprinkled in his fur, while short stubble hairs are a sign of licking

or scratching attempts to relieve irritation. Part the fur in several places and examine the skin beneath: it should be clean, pale, smooth and free of dandruff. Feel for any unusual lumps and bumps under the skin.

Having completed this overall check, take a closer look at specific parts of your dog's body, using the pictures below for reference.

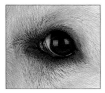

(Left) A dog's eyeballs should shine, and his pupils should be the same size. Squinting, excessive blinking and crying are all signs of eye discomfort.

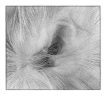

(Right) Healthy fur should be glossy and free from odour, with smooth skin beneath. Dandruff, scabs or greasy hair are signs of skin disorders.

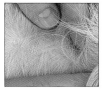

(Above) The inner surfaces of the ear flaps should be clean, smooth and slightly greasy. Ear-scratching, head-shaking or head-tilting all indicate possible problems.

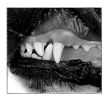

A dog's 42 adult teeth should be white, and the gums should be pink (excepting any pigmented areas).

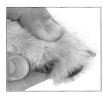

The claws should have rounded ends and a smooth outer surface. Matted fur or foreign bodies between the toes should be removed as soon as possible.

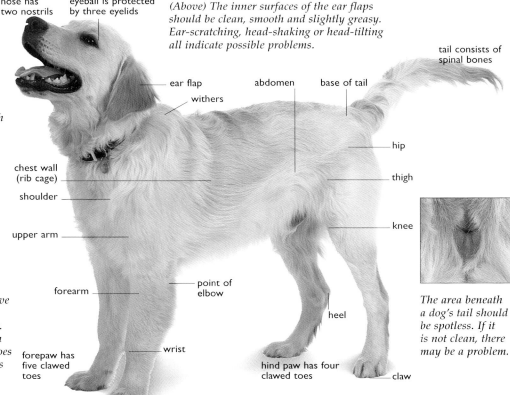

nose has two nostrils

eyeball is protected by three eyelids

ear flap

withers

abdomen

base of tail

tail consists of spinal bones

hip

chest wall (rib cage)

thigh

shoulder

upper arm

knee

forearm

point of elbow

heel

wrist

forepaw has five clawed toes

hind paw has four clawed toes

claw

The area beneath a dog's tail should be spotless. If it is not clean, there may be a problem.

Reference table of common symptoms

This reference table is a guide to the conditions covered in this book, and to some of the symptoms most commonly associated with them. The conditions are ordered by parts or systems of the body.

Use this table as a quick index to familiarize yourself with some of the most important symptoms relating to each condition, but avoid the temptation to use it as a home-diagnosis chart. If you are ever concerned or confused about anything to do with your dog's health or welfare, always contact your vet centre for advice.

EYE

EAR

MOUTH

DIGESTIVE SYSTEM

HEART

AIRWAYS

JOINTS, BONES AND LIGAMENTS

Lameness   44–5
(note: this is itself a symptom)
Arthritis   46–7
• swollen, painful joint
• lameness (often intermittent)
• stiffness, especially after rest
Bone fracture   48–9
• painful swelling over
  affected bone(s)
• obvious wound in some cases
• abnormal appearance to
  affected body part
• inability to use affected part of
  skeleton (e.g. broken leg carried)
Hip dysplasia   50–1
• swaying/bunny-hopping gait
• hindleg lameness/stiffness
Intervertebral-disc protrusion 52
• severe back/neck pain
• rigid stance/hunched posture
• paralysis/incontinence (in the
  worst cases)
Rupture of cranial cruciate
  ligament   53
• lameness
• characteristic toe-resting

SKIN AND COAT

Scratching and skin-nibbling 54
(note: this is itself a symptom)
Alopecia   55
• bald areas in coat
• hair thinning
Hypersensitivity reactions 56–7
• intense itchiness
• reddened skin
Fleas and other parasites 58–61
• itchiness (in most – but
  not all – cases)
• fleas, lice and ticks visible
  to naked eye
Pyoderma   62–3
• moist, smelly, inflamed skin sores

• pussy spots on skin
• inflamed swelling between toes
• smelly, inflamed skin folds
Seborrhoea   63
• skin flakiness
• greasy coat/hair loss
• inflamed, itchy skin
Claw conditions   64–5
• lameness
• overlong claws visible

KIDNEYS AND BLADDER

Cystitis   66
• frequent passing of small
  volumes of urine
• unexpected urination
  'accidents' indoors
• discomfort during urination
Chronic renal failure   67
• increased urine production
• increased drinking
• sickness/debility/weight loss
  (in advanced cases)
Urinary incontinence   68
• involuntary urine dribbling
  and soiling of bed

REPRODUCTIVE SYSTEM (FEMALE)

Pseudo-pregnancy   70–1
• breast enlargement and milk
  production
• nest-building behaviour
• over-attachment to objects
  such as toys
Pyometra   71
• 'mucky' vaginal discharge
  (not in all cases)
• general vague symptoms
  of ill-health
• increased thirst
• vomiting

REPRODUCTIVE SYSTEM (MALE)

Cryptorchidism   72
• less than two testicles in
  scrotum of sexually mature
  male dog
Prostate-gland disorders 73
• often no obvious symptoms
• constipation
• straining to urinate
• urinary incontinence
• blood or pus discharge from penis
• abdominal discomfort

OTHER IMPORTANT CONDITIONS

Cancer   74–5
• very variable symptoms
  depending on tumour type, size
  and location
• often general debility
Diabetes mellitus   76–7
• increased urination
• increased thirst
• increased appetite
• weight loss
Chronic liver disease   78
• reluctance to eat and weight loss
• depression and lethargy
• vomiting/diarrhoea
• jaundice (not in all cases)
Seizures ('fits')   79
• unconsciousness, tight jaw, fixed
  stare, leg-paddling, jaw-chomping
  for one or two minutes
Umbilical hernia   80
• swelling under skin at
  'tummy button'
Growing old (ageing) 80–1
• many symptoms
Obesity   82–3
• physical appearance
• ribs cannot be felt easily
• lethargy and tiredness on
  normal exercise

Common conditions

In this section you will find essential background information relating to some of the most common medical conditions suffered by dogs. This information is designed to complement the advice that you should obtain from the staff at your vet centre if your dog is ill and suffering from any of these conditions.

Eye

A dog's eyes are very complex biological cameras, and they and the tissues that surround them are vulnerable to numerous conditions. If there is any change at all in the appearance of your dog's eyes, or you suspect that his eyesight may be failing, you must take him to be examined by your vet as soon as possible. Any delay could result in him suffering from permanently defective sight. Before buying a puppy, find out from a vet centre whether or not your chosen breed is vulnerable to any hereditary eye conditions.

Cataract

A cataract is an opacity of the lens, or of the capsule that surrounds the lens, within a dog's eye. Depending on the cause, a cataract may affect just one or both of the eyes. Many – but not all – are progressive and worsen as time passes.

Causes

Hereditary cataracts are a well-known problem in certain breeds (see right), and are the result of an individual dog's genetic make-up. In some cases the cause of a cataract or cataracts is never discovered, but they may develop following injury to the lens or in association with other eye disorders. Total cataracts may develop in just a few weeks in a dog suffering from diabetes mellitus (see pages 76–7).

Is it serious?

This depends on the size and cause of the cataract, and on whether one or both of the eyes is affected. An acquired cataract in only one of a dog's eyes is unlikely to require treatment, unless there are sight problems from another cause that are affecting the other eye.

The most serious cataracts are the progressive type that affect both eyes. Many hereditary cataracts fall into this category. In a typical case the cataract or cataracts first appear when a puppy is a few weeks old, and will progress to cause total blindness in one to three years.

Dogs at risk

The following breeds of dog are just some of those that are currently known to suffer from hereditary cataracts, and this number is increasing all the time:
• American cocker spaniel
• Boston terrier
• Cavalier King Charles spaniel
• German shepherd
• Golden retriever
• Labrador retriever
• Large Munsterlander
• Miniature schnauzer
• Norwegian buhund
• Old English sheepdog
• Siberian husky
• Staffordshire bull terrier
• Standard poodle
• Welsh springer spaniel

COMMON SYMPTOMS

• In the early stages of a cataract, the only visible sign may be a slight greying of the lens (this may go undetected, or may be confused with nuclear sclerosis, an ageing condition of the lens).
• A dog with worsening cataracts may begin to bump into objects that have been moved from their normal location, and may become anxious in unfamiliar surroundings.
• An eye containing a lens with an advanced cataract will appear to have a white pupil.

Action

If you think that your dog could be suffering from a cataract or cataracts, arrange for your vet to examine him as soon as possible.

Your vet will begin by carrying out a complete clinical examination of your dog, before concentrating on his eyes. In order to look at the lenses of the eyes in detail, he or she will use an instrument called an ophthalmoscope (see page 91).

There are no specific tests that can be used to establish the quality of a dog's visual abilities, but your vet may set up an obstacle course for your dog to try.

If the signs of a cataract are not marked, but your vet is concerned that one may exist, he or she may recommend that your dog is seen by a veterinary eye specialist.

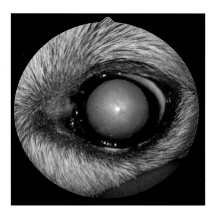

Using an ophthalmoscope (see page 91), a vet can carefully examine a dog's eye under magnification. Not all cataracts are as obvious as this one (above).

This Yorkshire terrier (below) has an advanced cataract in his left eye, which has caused total blindness in that eye.

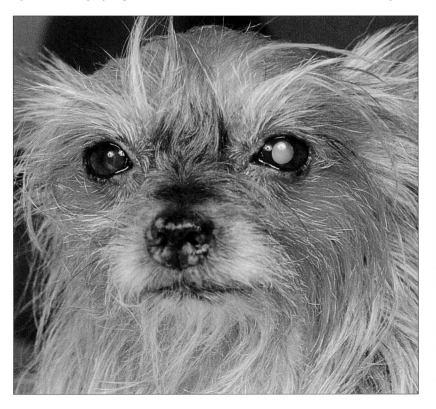

THE EYE SCHEME

Hereditary eye conditions in dogs will not disappear without careful screening. To this end, in the UK the British Veterinary Association, the International Sheepdog Society and the Kennel Club jointly run a screening programme known as the Eye Scheme.

Currently, the scheme covers 11 hereditary eye conditions of dogs, affecting 41 breeds. As well as cataracts, the conditions under scrutiny include certain serious problems of the retina, glaucoma (a build-up of fluid in the eye, causing tension within the eyeball), a condition called primary lens luxation (in which the lens 'falls' out of its normal position), and a number of congenital eye disorders that are identifiable in very young puppies.

A number of other hereditary eye conditions are also under investigation. It seems that, the more experts look for these conditions in different breeds of dog, the more problems they find.

If you intend to breed from a pure-bred dog, you should contact your vet centre to discuss your plans. Your vet will be able to arrange for your dog's eyes to be examined by one of over 40 vets authorized by the Eye Scheme. Your nearest authorized vet may not be local, but your visit will be very worthwhile.

The vet will examine your dog's eyes with special equipment, and will look for signs of hereditary or other eye conditions. You will be given a certificate with the results of the examination. The vet will also advise you of the results with regard to your breeding plans.

OUTSIDE THE UK

If you live outside the UK, ask your vet for details of any similar scheme that may be in operation in your country.

Treatment

There is no medical treatment for cataracts. It is possible to remove them by surgery, but this is a major and complex procedure that is only undertaken by vets with specialist knowledge and equipment.

The decision to go ahead with surgery should not be taken lightly, and you should consider your vet's advice very carefully. If surgery on your dog's eyes is to be attempted, it should be carried out before any problems that are associated with more advanced cataracts – such as inflammation – begin to occur.

Prevention

Nothing can be done to prevent cataracts. However, a dog who is suffering from hereditary cataracts should not be used for breeding.

A thorough eye examination by an authorized vet (see page 13) will reveal the presence of cataracts or any other inherited eye conditions. This is especially important for dogs of the following breeds, all of which are known (in the UK) to be susceptible to these conditions:

RESPONSIBLE BREEDING

To help prevent hereditary eye conditions from being passed from one generation to the next, it is important not to breed from dogs who are known sufferers. I would recommend that pure-bred dogs should undergo eye examinations before being used for breeding (see page 13), even if they belong to breeds not known to suffer from inherited eye conditions.

- American cocker, cocker, Tibetan, Cavalier King Charles and English springer spaniels
- Basenji
- Basset hound
- Bedlington, Boston, miniature bull, Sealyham, Staffordshire bull and smooth-haired and wire-haired fox terriers
- Border collie
- Briard
- Chesapeake Bay, golden and labrador retrievers
- Doberman pinscher
- Elkhound
- German shepherd
- Hungarian puli
- Irish setter
- Large Munsterlander
- Miniature schnauzer
- Miniature dachshund
- Norwegian buhund
- Old English sheepdog
- Parson Jack Russell
- Poodle
- Rough and smooth collies
- Rottweiler
- Shetland sheepdog
- Siberian husky
- Welsh corgi

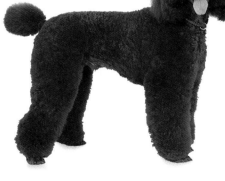

The standard poodle is prone to hereditary cataracts; these may be diagnosed before a dog is 18 months old.

Conjunctivitis

Conjunctivitis is an inflammation of the membrane that lines the inner surfaces of the eyelids and covers the exposed part of the eyeball (except the transparent cornea). Both sides of the third eyelid are also covered by this membrane. Conjunctivitis may be an acute or chronic condition affecting just one or both of the eyes.

Causes

Possible causes of conjunctivitis include bacterial, viral or fungal infections, allergies and physical irritation or damage resulting from the presence of foreign bodies such as thorns, grass seeds, other debris or even ingrowing eyelid hairs. The condition may also occur as a result of inadequate tear production.

Is it serious?

A case of mild and uncomplicated infectious conjunctivitis may not be particularly serious but, through scratching and rubbing at his face to relieve irritation, a dog may quickly cause further damage.

Conjunctivitis may also be associated with other underlying conditions of greater concern.

Dogs at risk

Any dog is at risk of developing conjunctivitis, although those dogs who tend to roam in areas of thick undergrowth may be more likely than dogs who are walked in areas of open country to pick up foreign bodies such as grass seeds or thorns in their eyes.

Breeds with eyelids that droop excessively may be particularly at risk from conjunctivitis caused by the presence of foreign bodies, while dogs with protruding eyes – such as the Pekinese – may be more vulnerable to eye trauma. Some breeds, including the German shepherd, seem to be at particular risk of suffering from certain types of non-infectious conjunctivitis.

Action

If you think that your dog may have conjunctivitis, but the signs appear mild and his eye (or eyes) is not causing obvious discomfort, bathe away any discharge around the eye using cotton wool soaked in plain water. Continue to monitor your dog's symptoms, and do not exercise him: he may find the wind in his face uncomfortable, and any eye discharge will also tend to attract dirt and debris.

Prevent your dog from having contact with any other dogs, as his condition could be infectious.

If the symptoms are worse after 24 hours, and the eye has become red and weepy, take your dog to be examined by your vet as soon as possible. However, if the symptoms remain mild, keep monitoring the situation. If your dog is not totally back to normal within three days, take him to your vet.

Your vet should give your dog a thorough examination to ensure that he is healthy in every other way before checking his eyes with an ophthalmoscope to gain a magnified, illuminated view of the external and internal features of the eyeballs (see page 91). After assessing the overall appearance of your dog's eyes, your vet may clean away any discharges to take a closer look at the conjunctival membranes and eyeball surfaces.

Your vet may also gently scrape a small sample of tissue from your dog's conjunctiva, for analysis in a laboratory (see page 93). This test may help to reveal the cause of the conjunctivitis, and will assist your vet in deciding on further treatment should your dog's condition not respond to routine therapy.

Treatment

If your vet can identify the cause of your dog's conjunctivitis during the initial consultation, he or she will institute appropriate therapy: for instance, removing a foreign body.

Even if the cause of the condition cannot be found at this stage, your vet is likely to choose a therapy regime from the following options:
• Antibiotic eye ointment or drops
• Anti-inflammatory eye ointment or drops
• Anti-inflammatory medications for administration by mouth (see pages 101–3).

Aftercare

Antibiotic eye ointment or drops should be continued for at least five days. You will need to give your dog his medication at home, so

This six-year-old German shepherd has a marked reddening and swelling of the membranes around his eye, associated with conjunctivitis.

make sure before leaving your vet centre that you know what to do, how much ointment or drops to use, and the daily timing of each dose (see also pages 101–3).

You will also need to keep your dog's eyes clean, using special eye-wipes or cotton wool dampened with plain water. To prevent him from scratching or rubbing at his eyes and causing further damage, you may need to fit him with an 'Elizabethan collar' (see page 108).

Prevention

You can help to prevent your dog suffering from conjunctivitis by gently wiping away any day-to-day discharge that may accumulate at the corners of his eyes, using moist face-wipes or cotton wool wetted with plain water.

It is sensible to avoid exposing your dog unnecessarily to other dogs with acute conjunctivitis, to minimize the risk of cross-infection.

COMMON SYMPTOMS

The precise cocktail of symptoms shown in a case of conjunctivitis will vary, depending on the cause.

However, the following are all symptoms that are most commonly associated with this condition:
• A reddened eye or eyes
• Increased tear production, or 'crying'

• Increased blinking
• Discharge from the corner of the eye (the discharge may be watery, or thick and gooey).
• Half-closed eyelids
• The dog may scratch at his eye or rub his face along the ground in an attempt to relieve the irritation that the conjunctivitis is causing him.

Corneal ulceration

The cornea is the transparent part of the front of the eyeball. It allows your dog to see out, and you to see into the deeper structures of his eye, such as the coloured iris that creates the shape of his pupil.

An ulcer forms when the smooth surface of the cornea is damaged.

Causes

There are a number of possible causes of corneal ulceration. These include a scratch or scrape on the cornea which may develop into an ulcer, ingrowing eyelid hairs rubbing across the cornea, or other eye conditions – such as inadequate tear production – that leave the cornea vulnerable to damage.

A foreign body becoming caught behind the eyelids or lodged in the cornea itself, a tumour on the eyelid or a bacterial infection may also result in a corneal ulcer.

Is it serious?

Yes. Any corneal ulcer is painful and, if left untreated, a small ulcer may spread across the cornea and deepen. Ulcers caused by bacteria called *Pseudomonas* are particularly aggressive, and are referred to as 'melting ulcers'. However, with prompt and appropriate treatment, many will heal quickly.

Some very deep ulcers require immediate surgery to patch and repair them as, left untreated, they may cause the cornea to rupture.

Dogs at risk

Corneal ulcers can occur in any dog, but members of breeds with bulbous eyes are most likely to damage their corneas. The boxer and Pembroke corgi seem to have an inherited predisposition to recurrent and persistent corneal

ulcers. Ageing dogs of all types also seem to be more prone to recurrent corneal ulceration.

Action

If your dog has a red, weeping eye that is causing obvious discomfort, contact your vet immediately.

After giving your dog a complete physical examination to check that he is otherwise well, your vet will examine his eyes thoroughly using an ophthalmoscope (see page 91).

To highlight a corneal ulcer, your vet may administer a dye called fluoroscein to your dog's cornea. The dye will adhere to an ulcer but will run off the undamaged surface of the cornea; it can be made more obvious by illuminating the eye with ultra-violet light.

If your vet confirms that an ulcer is present, he or she will carry out additional examinations, using the ophthalmoscope, to try to identify its cause prior to starting treatment.

Treatment

If caught early, most simple corneal ulcers heal without complications. An essential part of treating your

COMMON SYMPTOMS

The symptoms will depend on the cause and severity of the ulcer, but may include the following:
• Obvious discomfort
• Increased tear production
• Increased blinking
• Aversion to bright lights
• A red, inflamed eye
• The cornea may be slightly opaque and blue-grey in colour
• The conjunctiva may be swollen
• In a severe case, the edges of the ulcer may be visible .

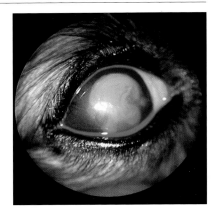

The fluoroscein dye administered to the eye of this three-year-old Pekinese will help to reveal ulceration of the cornea.

dog's condition will be for your vet to attend to any underlying cause: for instance, if a foreign body has been identified as the cause, your vet will remove it.

Your vet is also likely to begin treating your dog's injured eye with antibiotic eye ointment or drops, in order to keep bacteria at bay while the ulcer heals. You will need to continue administering this at home (see pages 102–3), and to keep your dog's eye clean. Do not exercise him off the lead until the ulcer has healed. To prevent your dog from further damaging his eye by rubbing at it, you may need to fit him with an 'Elizabethan collar' for a few days (see page 108).

If a corneal ulcer fails to heal despite the conventional treatment, further therapy may be needed; this may include any of the following:
• Surgical removal of loose corneal tissue around the ulcer.
• Chemical cauterization of the peeling ulcer edges.
• Surgery to create and fix a flap of healthy conjunctiva across the ulcer.

Epiphora

Tears produced by special glands within tissues around each eyeball are normally drained away through the tear duct, a small tube that links the inner corners of the upper and lower eyelid with the nose.

Epiphora occurs when normal tear drainage is impeded, causing tears to overflow on to the face.

Causes

A dog's tear duct, or the openings into it at the inner corner of the eye, may be malformed from birth, making the effective drainage of tears impossible.

Alternatively, the tear duct or its openings may seal up or become blocked later in the dog's life, due to problems such as infection of the tear duct, a foreign body, excessive mucus collection at the inner corner of the eyelids, or facial injury and subsequent scarring.

Is it serious?

Epiphora is not normally serious, unless an infection is involved.

Dogs at risk

Epiphora is most commonly seen in toy breeds, although any type of dog may suffer from the condition.

For tears to drain properly from the eye, the openings into the tear duct must be in contact with the tear film that covers the eyeball. In dogs with drooping eyelids, these openings may not be close enough to the eyeball to be able to drain tears effectively.

Action

If your dog has a longstanding weepy eye, or obvious tear-staining on his cheek, the effectiveness of his tear-drainage system should be assessed by your vet. Provided that the eye is not inflamed or painful this is not an emergency, but if there is inflammation you must make the appointment as soon as possible.

Your vet will begin by examining your dog's eye in detail, using an ophthalmoscope (see page 91). This will be to rule out the possibility that the overflow of tears may be due to overproduction: for instance, as a result of conjunctivitis (see pages 14–15) or corneal ulceration (see opposite), rather than poor drainage. To confirm this, your vet may place a special blotting paper behind your dog's eyelid, and will compare the rate of absorption of tears with figures for normal dogs.

During the examination your vet will look at the inner corners of the eyelids, to check whether the tear-duct openings are blocked. To assess the effectiveness of drainage, he or she may administer a dye called fluoroscein to the eye. If tear drainage is taking place, the dye will appear at your dog's nostril.

The dark fur-staining near the inner corners of this two-year-old miniature poodle's eyes is the result of epiphora.

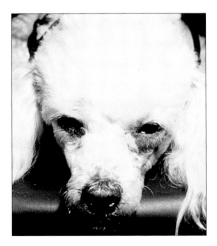

COMMON SYMPTOMS

Depending on its cause, epiphora may affect one or both eyes, and symptoms include the following:
• A constantly weeping eye
• A red, weeping eye, if the cause is an infection that has led on to conjunctivitis (see pages 14–15).
• Dark staining of the fur near the inner corner of the eye.

Treatment

In some cases, a blocked tear duct may be cleared by flushing saline or plain water through it, using a syringe with a very fine tube (called a canula) attached: this delicate procedure will be carried out with your dog either heavily sedated or anaesthetized (see pages 96–7).

If the epiphora is caused by an infection, your vet will prescribe antibiotic eye ointment or drops. In some cases, antibiotic injections and/or preparations to be given by mouth may be required. Surgery to correct defects in the tear-drainage system is rarely attempted.

Aftercare

If your vet prescribes antibiotics, you will need to administer them at home until the infection is cleared (see pages 101–3).

If the cause of the epiphora is untreatable, use special eye-wipes or cotton wool soaked in plain water to clean your dog's eyelids, as the accumulation of spilled tears may cause the skin around the eyes to become inflamed and infected.

Prevention

Cleaning your dog's eyes regularly should remove any dirt that could block his tear-duct openings.

Ear

A dog's ear is made up of three parts: the outer ear, including the ear flap, which 'collects' sounds and funnels them down to the ear drum; the middle ear, containing the ear bones (ossicles), which transmit the vibrations of the ear drum deeper into the ear; and the inner ear deep inside the skull, where vibrations originally created by the ear drum are converted into electrical signals that are transmitted to the brain. The most common ear condition of dogs is inflammation of the skin that lines the ear canal, or otitis externa.

Deafness

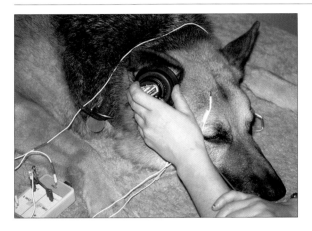

Special hearing tests for dogs with suspected hearing difficulties are now available from some veterinary hospitals. These tests employ equipment that was originally designed for use on people.

Deafness is not a condition in itself, but is a symptom of an underlying disorder. Temporary difficulties in hearing are fairly common in dogs, but permanent deafness is rare.

Deafness of any duration may be associated with problems in the transmission of sounds to the inner ear, or with disorders of the delicate parts of the inner ear that turn the sounds into electrical signals.

Problems with the nerves that carry these electrical signals away from the ear, or with the parts of the brain in which the signals are interpreted, may also occur.

COMMON SYMPTOMS

Many owners dismiss the signs of deafness, believing that their dogs are simply not responding as usual. These signs include the following:
• If one ear is affected, a dog may still hear fairly well but lose his ability to locate sources of sounds.
• He may not respond to sounds that normally provoke his interest.
• He may have difficulty in finding you when you call him on a walk.

Causes

Possible underlying causes of deafness include the following:
• Blockage of the ear canal by a foreign body, by debris associated with otitis externa (see pages 20–1), by fluid or by polyps (tumours).
• Damage to the ear drum.
• Damage to the ear bones, or a build-up of fluid, in the middle ear.
• Abnormalities in the inner ear associated with ageing.
• Anatomical abnormalities that occur during development.

Dogs at risk

Deafness is a known problem in young dalmations, as well as in the following breeds:
• Boston, bull and fox terriers
• Border and rough collies
• Cocker spaniel
• Doberman pinscher
• German shepherd
• Old English sheepdog

Action

If you suspect that your dog may have difficulty in hearing, carry out some very simple tests by checking his response to sounds of different pitch and intensity. If your dog does not respond as you would expect to these tests, take him to your vet.

Your vet will examine your dog's ears to rule out any obvious cause of the hearing difficulty, before carrying out further simple hearing tests. He or she may also arrange an electronic hearing test (if available).

Treatment

Your vet will remove any blockage of the ear canal, such as that caused by otitis externa (see pages 20–1).

Anatomical abnormalities cannot be cured. If your dog is confirmed as being permanently deaf, you can help him to cope with his condition: for example, it is perfectly possible to train a puppy using hand signals. You may also find it helpful to talk to other owners of deaf dogs.

Aural haematoma

An aural haematoma is a 'blood blister' of the ear flap. It occurs as a result of accumulation of 'bloody' fluid between the inner and outer skin surfaces of the ear flap, and around the rubbery cartilage sheet sandwiched between the skin.

Causes

It is thought likely that most aural haematomas are due to self-trauma resulting from ear irritation. In trying to relieve the discomfort of conditions such as otitis externa (see pages 20–1) or even fleas (see pages 56 and 58–9), a dog may damage his ear flap by banging it on a hard object while scratching, head-shaking vigorously or rubbing his face along the ground.

However, very recent studies offer a different story. They suggest that an aural haematoma may arise as a result of some kind of reaction of a dog's immune system, as the liquid in an aural haematoma is very watery and does not have the normal consistency of fresh blood.

Is it serious?

An aural haematoma in a dog is not usually a serious or life-threatening condition: a swollen and heavy ear flap may simply feel uncomfortable to a dog and look unsightly.

However, in many cases an aural haematoma can be surprisingly difficult to cure.

Dogs at risk

Any dog may suffer from an aural haematoma, but those with large, dangling ear flaps may be more prone to damaging them than dogs who have small, pricked ears. For reasons that are not understood, the golden retriever appears to be particularly susceptible.

Action

If you think that your dog may have an aural haematoma, your vet should examine him. This condition does not constitute an emergency, but prompt action is important as aural haematomas usually increase in size as time passes, and become more difficult to treat.

An aural haematoma is easy to identify through examination. Your vet will also look down your dog's ear holes with an instrument called an otoscope (see page 91) to check for underlying conditions. A full examination of the rest of his body should reveal the presence of any irritating skin parasites such as fleas (see pages 58–9).

Treatment

There are a number of treatment options. The most appropriate technique will depend on the size, shape and precise location of your dog's haematoma. Your vet may carry out any of the following:

Aspiration of the bloody fluid within the haematoma • In this procedure, the fluid is drawn out using a syringe and needle, and is followed immediately by an

---

COMMON SYMPTOMS

• An aural haematoma may be visible as a soft swelling with a smooth outline (this may be small, or may involve the whole ear flap).
• An affected ear flap will be heavier than normal, so the dog may hold it in an unusual position.
• An underlying condition that affects the skin or ear will cause the dog to show other symptoms, such as head-shaking.

---

injection of a powerful anti-inflammatory preparation into the cavity. Alternatively, the injection may be given one or two days after drainage.

Drainage • An open drainage tube may be inserted through the haematoma and left in place for as long as three weeks in order to empty its contents.

Opening of the haematoma • Under a general anaesthetic (see pages 96–7), the haematoma is opened and its contents flushed out. Your vet will then insert sutures right through the ear flap to clamp the skin that covered the haematoma to the underlying cartilage. The wound is left open so that any fluid can escape.

In numerous cases, more than one attempt is required to cure an aural haematoma. It is difficult to ensure that – once the fluid is removed – the skin adheres to the ear-flap cartilage: the process is rather like trying to stick two wet pieces of adhesive tape together!

Aftercare

If the haematoma has been opened and stitched, your dog may have his ear bandaged to the top of his head; if a drainage tube has been inserted, he may need to wear an 'Elizabethan collar' (see page 108). In either case, his fur will become soiled with discharge. Applying petroleum jelly will help any fluid to run off; your vet or a nurse will show you how to clean the wound.

You may have to administer antibiotics and/or painkillers.

Prevention

Always seek prompt attention for your dog if he shows signs of ear irritation, such as head-shaking.

Otitis externa

One part of a dog's skin that is all too often out of sight and out of mind is the small part that lines his ear canals – that is, until something goes wrong with it.

Otitis externa is inflammation of the skin lining the ear canal, and is one of the most common of all conditions of dogs treated by vets.

Causes

The anatomy of a dog's ear may cause or contribute to otitis externa. The skin that lines the ear canal produces wax as a protective barrier, and the loss of dried wax through head-shaking and the dog's ear movements normally matches the production of the wax.

The evaporation of water from the wax is an essential part of its removal and relies on adequate ventilation of the ear canal, but the structure of the ears of some dogs (see below, right) hinders this process. Excessive wax in the ear

canal irritates the skin that lines it, stimulating it to produce yet more wax. The result is the perfect environment for normally harmless bacteria and fungi living within the ear to multiply, and, in doing so, to cause inflammation.

Other common causes of otitis externa include ear mites (see opposite, below), a foreign body lodged in the ear canal, bacterial or fungal infections, or generalized skin problems such as atopy (see page 57).

Is it serious?

If caught early, no. However, if it is left untreated otitis externa can become a chronic condition, resulting

Your vet will use an otoscope to examine your dog's ears in detail (see also page 91).

COMMON SYMPTOMS

Otitis externa may involve one or both ears. If you suspect that your dog's ears are irritating him, gently rub his face under his ear holes and watch for his reaction. If he scratches at your hand, makes whining noises of delight or yelps in discomfort, he is likely to have a problem.

Other symptoms of otitis externa include the following:
- A smelly ear
- Discharge from the ear
- Vigorous head-shaking and/or ear-scratching.
- Head-rubbing on the ground or against objects.
- Resentment of handling or fussing around the ear.

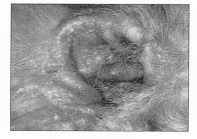

A dog with severe otitis externa will be in considerable discomfort. This dog's ear is likely to need aggressive treatment for many weeks.

- Reddened skin at the ear hole (the inner ear flap may also be affected).

in some cases in ulceration of the lining of the ear canal, rupture of the ear drum and the subsequent involvement of the inner ear.

Permanent damage to the ear-canal lining, caused by a delay in carrying out appropriate treatment, may also make another episode of otitis externa more likely.

Dogs at risk

Dogs of breeds with unnatural ear conformation are often affected by recurrent otitis externa. For instance, the cocker spaniel has heavy, hanging ear flaps that inhibit ventilation of the ear canals, while the poodle has very narrow ear canals with folded linings that trap wax. The German shepherd and dachshund seem to produce more wax than most other dogs. Breeds with very hairy ears are more prone to wax build-up in their ear canals.

Dogs who swim on a frequent basis or who live in very humid environments are also at risk.

Action

If you think your dog may have otitis externa, or he is showing any of the other symptoms described, you should arrange for him to be examined by your vet as soon as possible. If he is head-shaking and scratching frantically, he may well have a foreign body in his ear canal, and you should contact your vet centre immediately.

Do not attempt to clean away any discharge from your dog's ear or ears before taking him for his appointment, as your vet may be able to gain valuable clues as to the cause of the problem by examining and testing this discharge.

Otitis externa may be associated with some other, more generalized, illnesses, so your vet should start by giving your dog a thorough clinical examination. He or she will try to look down his ear canals with an otoscope (see page 91), but may not be able to see very much because of the build-up of wax. Ear mites (see below, right) can also be difficult to spot, as they will hide under pieces of wax as soon as the light from the otoscope reaches them.

If the cause of your dog's otitis externa is unclear but there seems to be an infection present, your vet may elect to take a sample of any discharge for laboratory analysis. This should identify any organisms involved, and the medications that will bring them under control.

Treatment

Topical medicine • In a mild case of otitis externa, the use of ear ointment or drops is usually effective. Your dog may need more than one kind of topical medicine: for instance, if he has ear mites he will need a drug to kill the mites, but your vet may also use anti-inflammatory drugs to relieve irritation. If infection is either a causal or a contributing factor, antibiotic ear drops or ointment, or anti-fungal drugs, may be required. Otitis externa can be very painful, so your vet may prescribe painkillers.

Ear syringing • In a chronic case, the build-up of wax and other debris may be so severe that the ear canal needs to be washed out for the cause to be identified, or for the presence of a foreign body to be ruled out. A clean ear will also allow medicines better access to the site where they are needed. If your dog's ear is very dirty and impacted, it may need to be syringed out under an anaesthetic (see pages 96–7).

Reconstructive surgery • Creating better ear-canal ventilation may be the only way of preventing repeated bouts of otitis externa in certain dogs.

Aftercare

At home, you must administer prescribed ear ointments or drops, and perhaps medicines by mouth (see pages 101–2); treatment may continue for two weeks or more. You will also have to clean away any discharge on your dog's ear flap or around his ear hole. He will need regular check-ups by your vet.

Prevention

If you have a dog with very hairy ear holes, regular plucking of the hair may help to improve his ear-canal ventilation (consult your vet before attempting this yourself).

I would not advocate the routine use of ear-cleaning solutions on most normal dogs, as creating a moist environment within the ear canal may encourage the build-up of wax rather than its removal. If your dog has sensitive ears, try to keep him out of stagnant water.

Look at and sniff your dog's ear holes as part of his routine health-checks (see pages 8–9). You will quickly learn what his ears look like and how they smell when they are healthy, and will then be able to spot any problem quickly.

EAR MITES

Ear mites (*Otodectes cyanotis*) are tiny creatures that live in the ears of dogs, cats and other meat-eating animals. They feed on skin flakes and debris. Your dog is most likely to pick up ear mites through contact with an already infested dog or cat. Many cats seem to tolerate these creatures living in their ears very well, and an apparently healthy cat may pass them on to your dog while showing no symptoms.

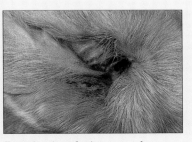

Ear mites in a dog's ear canals may produce characteristic brown wax and cause a great deal of irritation.

Mouth

Dogs tend to investigate the world around them with their mouths. As a result of this headlong approach, it is hardly surprising that oral injuries – especially broken teeth, bleeding gums and impaled foreign bodies (see pages 34–5) – are commonplace.

Gum disease – or periodontal disease, to use its proper name – is a largely preventable problem that is suffered sooner or later by the vast majority of dogs. If you do not already brush your dog's teeth, turn to pages 24–5 to find out why doing this regularly is so important.

Apical abscess

An apical abscess is a pocket of bacterial infection at the tip, or apex, of a tooth root. The tooth roots most commonly affected are generally those of the carnassial teeth in the upper jaw: these are the largest teeth in a dog's mouth, and are used for shearing and cutting food. Apical abscesses involving these teeth are often referred to as malar abscesses.

Although an affected tooth root may be very obviously damaged in many cases, the tooth itself appears normal at first sight.

COMMON SYMPTOMS

• The first sign of an apical abscess involving an upper carnassial tooth is often a discrete swelling on the face, just in front of the eye.
• An affected dog may become head-shy, and may be less keen than usual to chew on hard objects. However, although the condition is presumably painful, most dogs continue to eat.

This dog is suffering from an abscess affecting the upper carnassial tooth.

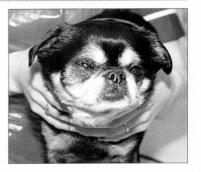

Causes

An apical abscess may develop following the fracture of a tooth and exposure of the sensitive pulp cavity to contamination.

Another possible cause of the condition is the concussion that occurs during chewing of hard objects, such as bones. This may interfere with the blood supply to an affected tooth root, allowing bacteria to become established.

Is it serious?

Once an apical abscess has formed, it is very unlikely to resolve itself without appropriate therapy. If it is left untreated, a malar abscess may burst and discharge its contents of pus out on to the dog's face and possibly into his eye, or internally into the nose. However, emergency treatment is not normally required.

Dogs at risk

Any kind of dog may be at risk of suffering from an apical abscess, although some vets believe that mongrels may be more vulnerable than their pure-bred cousins.

Most affected dogs are middle-aged or older animals.

Action

If your dog suddenly develops a small swelling on his face, you should make an appointment for him to be examined by your vet. If the abscess bursts before then, clean up any discharge using warm, salty water, and try to bring your appointment forward.

The signs of an apical abscess may be obvious, but your vet may also take an X-ray picture of your dog's jaw (see page 92) to confirm the condition.

Treatment

A course of antibiotics may help to control the infection, but an abscess may quickly recur once treatment is stopped unless the source of the infection is removed.

Your vet may suggest extracting the affected tooth. However, if it is important for some reason to save the tooth, your vet may decide to refer your dog to a dentistry specialist, to establish whether carrying out root-canal procedures may be appropriate.

Aftercare

Following the initial treatment, carried out either at your vet centre or by the dentistry specialist, you may need to administer prescribed antibiotics to your dog at home (see pages 101–2). He may also be given painkillers to relieve discomfort.

Prevention

Regular chewing of hard materials such as stones and bones may wear down or break a dog's teeth (see right), and may predispose him to suffering from apical abscesses.

You should try to avoid this by encouraging your dog to chew on more malleable objects, such as well-designed, tough rubber toys.

BROKEN AND WORN-DOWN TEETH

The pulp cavity inside a dog's tooth is very sensitive, and may be exposed if the tooth is broken. If left untreated, contamination of the cavity may result in the tooth root becoming loose or infected. Capping the cavity may save the tooth from further disease and is most effective if carried out within hours, so a broken tooth should be considered an emergency.

A tooth that has been worn down by excessive grinding may appear to have an open pulp cavity, as there may well be a brown mark at its centre. However, this is actually a natural repair carried out by the tooth itself.

Pharyngitis (and tonsillitis)

The pharynx is the area at the back of a dog's throat that contains his two tonsils: the special tissues that form part of his immune system.

Pharyngitis is inflammation of the lining of the pharynx; tonsillitis is inflammation of the part of the pharynx that contains the tonsils.

Causes

Some of the potential causes of these conditions are as follows:
• The mouth is a common route by which infectious organisms enter the body, and both pharyngitis and tonsillitis are often a result of viral infections that also affect other parts of the body.
• Localized pharyngitis may be caused by bacterial infection due to a foreign body impaled in the lining of the pharynx (see pages 34–5).
• The pharynx and tonsils may become infected as a result of the symptoms of other conditions,

such as vomiting (see pages 28–9) or chronic coughing.
• Severe periodontal disease (see pages 24–5) may cause bacterial infection, and the subsequent inflammation of the pharynx.

Is it serious?

In most cases, no. In some dogs, particularly those with shortened muzzles such as the pug and British bulldog, the inflamed pharynx and enlarged tonsils may restrict an already compromised airflow and contribute to breathing problems.

Dogs at risk

Pharyngitis may occur in any dog of any age. Tonsillitis is common in young dogs, especially of small breeds, and may be associated with the development of their oral immune-defence mechanisms.

Action

If you suspect pharyngitis, arrange for your dog to see your vet. In the meantime, do not offer him hard foods, remove his collar indoors and avoid exercising him.

Your vet will look for the typical reddening caused by inflammation of the pharynx lining and tonsils. The tonsils may also be swollen, and your dog may have a raised temperature associated with a fever.

Treatment

In most cases, antibiotics quickly control bacterial infection, provided that any obvious cause – such as a foreign body – has been removed. Your vet may also prescribe mild painkillers to relieve discomfort.

Aftercare

The initially painful period of three to five days is usually followed by complete recovery in about a week.

As well as administering the prescribed medicines to your dog, you should liquidize his food (or add water) for the first few days, to make it easier for him to swallow. You should also avoid exercising him unnecessarily.

Prevention

Brushing your dog's teeth regularly (see page 25) will help to reduce the bacterial burden in his mouth.

COMMON SYMPTOMS

• Retching, as if attempting to clear the throat.
• Coughing
• Difficulty in swallowing
• Reluctance to eat – especially hard foods – despite being hungry (in some cases).

WARNING

Throwing sticks for your dog could result in splinters becoming stuck in his pharynx; chewing the wood may also damage his gums. When you play with your dog, throw a ball or a safe toy such as a special dog 'frisbee' instead.

Periodontal disease

Periodontal disease literally means disease of the tissues that surround and support the teeth. It is the most common oral condition suffered by dogs. For example, in the UK the majority of dogs over two years old are thought to suffer from this condition to some degree.

Causes

This condition is the result of events that will have been going on in your dog's mouth since the day his teeth first came through.

The outer surface of the teeth is made of enamel. In a young dog, it is smooth. Day by day, the teeth become covered in a material called plaque, which consists mainly of bacteria, but the action of chewing wipes this away to some extent.

Plaque is soft in texture, but it quickly hardens to produce calculus, or tartar. Unlike enamel, calculus is rough, so plaque is more

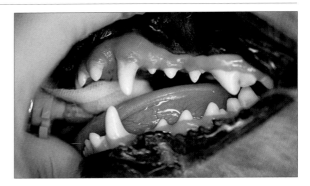

This young adult dog has healthy gums that are pink, but not red and inflamed. His teeth are clean and smooth, and he does not have bad breath.

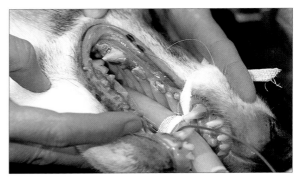

This older dog has been anaesthetized (see pages 96–7) so that his vet can carry out treatment for periodontal disease. The dog's teeth are covered with rough calculus and his gums are seriously inflamed. He may well lose some teeth.

COMMON SYMPTOMS

- Bad breath (a healthy dog's breath may not smell as sweet as yours, but should not be offensive)
- Yellow/brown marks on the teeth at gum edges, especially on the upper carnassial tooth and the first molar tooth. These 'marks' will be rough-looking crusts in advanced cases
- Reddened gum edges
- Receding gums and exposed tooth roots, especially of the canine teeth
- Difficulty in chewing food
- Reluctance to eat
- Drooling saliva (this may be blood-tinged)
- Mouth pain, shown by the dog pawing at his mouth or rubbing his face along the ground.

---

difficult to remove from it. The bacteria in plaque irritate the gum and cause it to swell: a condition called gingivitis. As the gum grows more inflamed, other damaging bacteria become involved and the gum may start to recede.

Finally, the attachments of the tooth are weakened, and it becomes loose. The process can take several years to complete, but is reversible in the early stages.

Is it serious?

Advanced periodontal disease is painful, and is likely to result in loss of teeth. A calculus-covered tooth may act as a reservoir of infection, and bacteria may find their way via the blood to other organs such as the heart, kidneys, liver and lungs, where they could cause disease.

Dogs at risk

All dogs are at risk of periodontal disease, although particular factors may promote its development. For instance, a retained deciduous tooth (see page 26), or overcrowded teeth in dogs with small mouths (such as those with short muzzles and flat faces), may trap food. A diet of soft, 'sticky' food may promote plaque retention, while chewing bones, stones and wood may damage the gums and lead to infection.

Action

If you suspect periodontal disease, take your dog for a check-up with your vet. Even if you have a young dog, or an older individual with gleaming white teeth, you should incorporate regular tooth-brushing into his routine care (see opposite).

Your vet will examine your dog's mouth for the obvious signs of periodontal disease, checking the gums for signs of inflammation and possibly also using a disclosing solution to reveal any build-up of plaque on the teeth.

Treatment

The aim of treatment is to remove plaque and calculus to give the supporting structures of the teeth a healthier environment. In mild cases, the only treatment required may be the removal of soft plaque through tooth-brushing (see right).

If calculus is present, it will need to be removed by descaling, carried out under a general anaesthetic (see pages 96–7). This involves the use of ultrasonic, vibrating instruments that literally shake the deposits from the teeth. The teeth are then polished so that their surfaces are less attractive to plaque.

In an advanced case, it may be impossible to tell how badly a tooth's attachments are affected by periodontal disease because the tooth is covered by calculus. If descaling shows the attachments to be seriously damaged, your vet may need to extract the tooth.

In exceptional cases, a diseased tooth may be saved by advanced dental-surgery techniques.

Aftercare

The benefits of treatment to your dog will soon be lost if you do not continue with home dental care.

Prevention

Plaque must be regularly removed before it hardens into tartar and damages the gums. This can be achieved in the following ways:

Daily tooth-brushing • This will remove plaque. It is an unusual and an unnatural experience for a dog to have his teeth brushed,

---

BRUSHING YOUR DOG'S TEETH

Although he will lose his milk teeth, you should start brushing a puppy's teeth as soon as you bring him home: the sooner he becomes used to this, the better.

TOOTH-BRUSHING EQUIPMENT
• Toothpaste: special palatable toothpastes are available for dogs. Do not use human toothpaste, as most dogs seem to find frothy mint paste in their mouths unpleasant, and it is best not swallowed on a regular basis.

• Although there are toothbrushes made especially for dogs, a good-quality human brush with firm bristles is ideal. Ask at your vet centre about the size of brush to use.

• Antiseptic rinses/sprays: these are particularly useful in dogs who suffer badly from gingivitis.

BRUSHING TECHNIQUE
At first, accustom your dog to the feel of the brush by holding his mouth closed and placing the brush in the pouch formed by his cheek for several seconds. Reward him for staying calm. Each day, keep the brush in his mouth a little longer, and begin to move it about. When your dog is used to this, start to brush the outsides of his back teeth: dip the brush in water, then hold it at 45 degrees to the teeth and move it in small circles. Then move on to the more sensitive area at the front of the mouth. Once he is happy about brushing with water, start using toothpaste.

Ask your vet or a veterinary nurse to demonstrate tooth-brushing, and for advice on the best dental-care products.

---

but it is a procedure to which the majority of dogs quickly become accustomed.

Diet • In general, dogs who are fed entirely on soft foods appear to suffer more periodontal disease than those offered foods that encourage chewing. It may help to offer your dog large pieces of hard, raw vegetables and tough, fibrous meat such as heart, ox skirt, cheek muscle or bovine trachea to chew on once a week, but do not overdo this or you may upset the balance of his diet.

Chewing bones devoid of meat will be of no benefit, and may harm your dog's teeth and gums.

Toys and chews • Special 'dental' toys and chews are claimed by the makers to control periodontal disease; one type has grooves in it for filling with toothpaste. There are also nylon toys in many shapes and sizes. These may be useful supplements but are not alternatives to tooth-brushing. Offering your dog a 'rawhide' chew once or twice a week may also help.

Retained deciduous tooth

Dogs, like humans, have two sets of teeth during their lives. A set of 28 deciduous, or 'milk', teeth begins to erupt when a puppy is between two and four weeks old. Then, from about 12 weeks of age onwards, the roots of these teeth gradually begin to disappear, and a set of 42 larger, permanent teeth begins to emerge.

If something disrupts the process by which a deciduous tooth is shed, its permanent replacement will be forced to grow in an abnormal direction. The deciduous tooth may fall out under pressure and the permanent tooth may come back into line, but in many cases the deciduous tooth remains in place and the permanent tooth erupts in the wrong position.

This condition may affect just one or a number of teeth.

Causes

The cause of a retained deciduous tooth, or teeth, is not known, but it may be a hereditary condition.

Is it serious?

Permanent damage may be caused to the jaw due to the misalignment of teeth. A canine tooth in the lower jaw that is forced to grow inwards because of a retained tooth could also puncture the roof of the mouth, creating an open hole into the nose.

At the very minimum, a retained deciduous tooth or teeth will put a dog at greater risk of suffering from early periodontal disease (see pages 24–5).

Dogs at risk

This condition appears to affect certain families of dogs, so a puppy with a parent who has suffered from a retained deciduous tooth or teeth may be affected in turn.

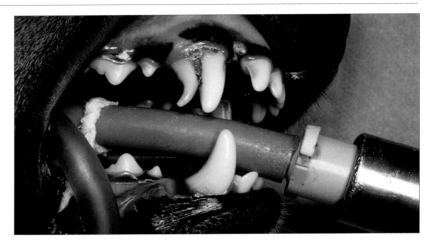

Action

If you have a puppy, you should regularly examine his mouth as part of his routine health-checks (see pages 8–9). If you think that he may have a deciduous and a permanent tooth lying side by side, or if he shows any symptoms associated with this condition, you should take him to see your vet. In most cases this is not an emergency, but you should not delay your visit by more than a few days.

Your vet will confirm whether your dog has a retained deciduous

COMMON SYMPTOMS

- The deciduous and permanent teeth may be obvious, especially in the case of canine teeth.
- The dog may be unable to close his mouth properly, as the teeth cannot interlock normally.
- Blood-tinged saliva may be present, caused by damage from an abnormally angled tooth.
- Reddened gums may be caused by infection, resulting from food being trapped between the teeth.

This dog has retained his upper right deciduous canine tooth; the permanent tooth has been forced to emerge in front of it. The deciduous tooth is being removed under a general anaesthetic.

tooth by carrying out a close and careful examination of his mouth.

Treatment

The retained deciduous tooth must be removed as soon as possible, to give the erupting permanent tooth the best chance of growing in the correct position.

Aftercare

After the extraction, you must administer any medication – such as painkillers – that your vet may prescribe (see pages 101–2). You should also liquidize (or add extra water to) your dog's food for a few days while his gums recover.

Prevention

Until we understand more about the causes of this condition, it is wise to avoid breeding from a dog who has suffered from a retained deciduous tooth as a puppy.

Undershot and overshot bite

The four parts of a dog's jaw (the upper and lower jaw on the right and left sides) grow independently. However, by interlocking with each other, the upper and lower teeth act as a kind of splint when the mouth is closed, ensuring that the upper and lower jaw grow forwards at the same rate.

In dogs with naturally shaped faces, this close alignment between the teeth of the lower and upper jaw allows the individual teeth to cut and shear food properly.

If, for some reason, the teeth do not line up as they should, a dog's upper jaw may end up being longer or shorter than his lower jaw. If the upper jaw overhangs the lower jaw, the dog is described as having an 'overshot' bite; if the lower jaw is longer than his upper jaw, he will have an 'undershot' bite.

Due to human interference in the breeding of dogs, an undershot jaw is considered to be normal in dogs of certain breeds that have flattened faces (the so-called brachycephalic breeds), such as the bulldog. This is in fact very unnatural, and these dogs are prone to other conditions of the mouth as a result.

COMMON SYMPTOMS

The symptoms exhibited by a dog with an undershot or an overshot jaw will depend on the severity of his condition, but he may show the following:
- An abnormal muzzle profile
- Spilling food when eating
- Difficulty in chewing
- Other signs that are associated with periodontal disease (see pages 24–5), to which dogs with this condition are very prone.

Causes

Trauma to a dog's mouth during puppyhood, or retained deciduous teeth (see opposite) may prevent a dog with a naturally shaped face from being able to close his mouth properly. As a result, his teeth will not interlock together in the correct way. Dogs of brachycephalic breeds are genetically destined to suffer from an undershot bite.

Is it serious?

The seriousness of this condition depends on its severity. Amazingly, most dogs with jaw abnormalities of this kind seem to be able to cope extremely well with their disability, as individuals of the brachycephalic breeds demonstrate.

Dogs at risk

Any kind of dog is at risk. All those of the brachycephalic breeds will suffer from an undershot bite to a greater or lesser degree.

Action

When choosing a young puppy of any breed (other than one of a brachycephalic breed, or cross-breed), you should check that he is able to close his mouth properly and that his upper front incisor teeth just overlap the lower ones when his mouth is closed.

If you are in any doubt about the bite of a particular puppy or dog whom you are interested in taking on as a pet, you should ask at your vet centre for advice.

Treatment

In most cases no treatment will be attempted, but corrective surgery may be an option to be considered in exceptional circumstances.

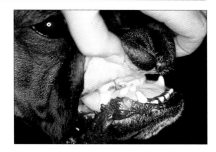

The undershot jaw of this boxer is an anatomical abnormality, but is accepted as being 'normal' for the breed.

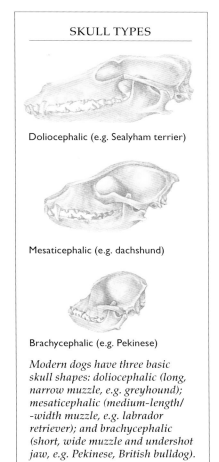

SKULL TYPES

Doliocephalic (e.g. Sealyham terrier)

Mesaticephalic (e.g. dachshund)

Brachycephalic (e.g. Pekinese)

Modern dogs have three basic skull shapes: doliocephalic (long, narrow muzzle, e.g. greyhound); mesaticephalic (medium-length/-width muzzle, e.g. labrador retriever); and brachycephalic (short, wide muzzle and undershot jaw, e.g. Pekinese, British bulldog).

Digestive system

A dog's digestive system works as a remarkable food processor that breaks down the food before it is absorbed through the bowel wall and used by the body. Any condition that adversely affects the way that this system functions may have serious consequences.

Vomiting and diarrhoea are perhaps the most common digestive-system problems to be suffered by dogs. They are in fact considered by vets to be symptoms of other conditions, but are included here as specific conditions as this is how most owners perceive them.

Vomiting

Vomiting is a reflex muscular act that results in the forceful ejection of a dog's stomach contents (and sometimes also some of the small-intestinal contents) through the mouth. It should not be confused with regurgitation, which – despite causing a similar end result in some cases – is a much more passive and relaxed act. Vomiting may occur as a sudden and severe condition, or as a low-grade, chronic complaint.

The majority of dogs tend to be fairly indiscriminate about what they will chew and swallow, but, fortunately, they have a highly sensitive vomit reflex that helps to reject inappropriate items from their digestive systems. As a result, occasional vomiting is common in many normal, healthy dogs.

Causes

A dog may vomit for many reasons, including the following:
• A sudden change in his diet, or other diet-related problems such as scavenging and ingesting unusual or spoiled food items, including grass or decaying garbage.
• An alteration in the chemical composition of the blood: this may be associated with a number of conditions, including chronic renal failure (see page 67), diabetes mellitus (see pages 76–7), liver disease (see page 78) and heatstroke (see page 123), or with a serious bacterial infection in a part of the

body, such as pyometra in a bitch (see page 71).
• A stomach disorder, including a foreign body (see pages 34–5), a stomach ulcer, stomach cancer or a life-threatening condition known as gastric dilatation/torsion, in which the stomach distends with gas and may then twist.
• An intestinal disorder, such as a parasitic-worm infestation (see pages 32–4), constipation (see page 37) or certain types of diarrhoea.
• A nervous reaction resulting from fear or stress.
• Motion sickness, or any other condition that may affect the dog's sense of balance such as some forms of ear disease.
• A specific infection such as distemper or canine parvovirus (see page 84).
• Trauma to the head.

Is it serious?

Vomiting can be life-threatening, but the seriousness of an individual case will depend on the underlying cause of the vomiting, on the time that has elapsed since its onset and on its frequency.

Anything other than sporadic and occasional vomiting – which is known to be associated with a dog's scavenging activities – should be considered potentially serious.

Severe, frequent vomiting should be considered an emergency, due to its major effects on body chemistry.

Dogs at risk

All dogs are at risk of vomiting.

Action

If your dog vomits, keep him indoors, observe him carefully and do not offer him anything to eat or drink for at least four hours. If he goes to the toilet, check whether he is also suffering from diarrhoea (see pages 30–1). If he does not vomit again, treat him as normal.

If your dog does vomit again within four hours, withhold food for a further 24 hours, but offer him a few laps of fresh water every 30 minutes. (Calculate the minimum number of millilitres of water that he should drink in the 24-hour period by multiplying his weight in kilogrammes by 40.) If he continues to vomit, cannot keep any water down or shows other signs of being unwell, such as lethargy, contact your vet straight away.

If your dog remains well in himself and does not vomit again within the 24-hour period, offer him unrestricted access to water, but make sure that he does not drink excessively at one sitting. Feed him a small, highly digestible, low-fat, low-fibre meal of cooked rice, pasta or potato, with a little hard-boiled egg, fish or chicken. Better still, offer a commercially prepared food formulated for dogs with digestive disturbances (see page 104).

COMMON SYMPTOMS

Vomiting may be the only – or the major – symptom of some conditions such as acute gastritis (inflammation of the stomach wall) due to mild food poisoning from eating spoiled food. In other conditions, such as certain bowel disorders, vomiting may occur in combination with other symptoms, including diarrhoea (see pages 30–1).

The act of vomiting involves three recognized phases:
• Nausea: as this phase begins, the dog may start to look concerned, and will salivate excessively, lick his lips and swallow repeatedly.

• Retching: the stomach begins to contract and changes occur in the dog's throat that prevent him from inhaling, and vomit will soon appear in his mouth. Forceful breathing movements are characteristic of this second phase.
• Vomiting: this final stage involves the co-ordinated movement of the dog's diaphragm and abdominal-wall muscles, resulting in a heaving action. This action puts great pressure on the stomach, and forces its contents up the oesophagus and out through the dog's mouth.

Continue to offer your dog small meals of this type every four hours during the day. If he remains well and does not vomit again, you can gradually add increasing amounts of his normal food over the next two days. By the end of the two days, he should be completely back on to his normal dietary regime.

If your dog needs veterinary treatment, your vet's aim will be to identify and treat any underlying cause of the vomiting, to replace any lost fluids, and to control the vomiting episodes so that they do not complicate the condition.

In an attempt to find the cause, your vet will examine your dog and will ask you about the timing of vomiting episodes and the nature of the vomit produced. Further diagnostic tests may include blood tests, X-ray and ultrasound investigations, and examinations with an endoscope (see pages 91–3).

Treatment

This will depend on the severity of the vomiting, and on any identified cause. Many cases of vomiting can be managed using medicines, but others – such as obstructions due to foreign bodies – may need surgery.

A case of sudden and severe vomiting will require intensive therapy to control the symptoms and to treat the effects of repeated vomiting on body chemistry. If a specific cause is not identified, treatment is likely to be based on a regime that includes the following:
• Nothing given by mouth for 24 to 48 hours.
• Immediate treatment with fluids given via an intravenous drip (see page 95), until the dog is able to take in sufficient water by mouth.
• Drugs to control the nausea and the vomiting episodes, to give the dog's digestive system a rest and to prevent further loss of fluids.

(Note: in most acute cases, the above regime will be initiated at the same time as investigations into the cause of the vomiting are carried out. If a cause is subsequently identified, additional treatment may be implemented.)

Your dog may need to remain at your vet centre as an

Do not feed your dog just before travelling with him in the car.

in-patient for these investigations or for treatment, particularly if he is very unwell.

Aftercare

When your dog comes home, you must administer his medicines and implement the dietary advice that you are given. Do not exercise him until he has fully recovered.

Prevention

It may be impossible to prevent many causes of vomiting, but the following are sensible precautions:
• Keep your dog's vaccinations up to date (see page 85).
• Regularly treat him for parasitic intestinal worms (see pages 32–4).
• Discourage him from scavenging.
• Do not feed him just before exercising him or travelling.
• Do not make any sudden changes to his diet, but gradually mix in a new food with the old one.
• Discourage your dog from bolting his food by spreading it thinly or by placing a large stone in his bowl so that he cannot excavate huge mouthfuls.
• If your dog has a big appetite, split up his food into two or more daily meals.

Diarrhoea

Diarrhoea is most obvious as the production of very watery faeces, although a dog who is defecating more frequently or is producing larger volumes of faeces than is normal may also be described as suffering from diarrhoea.

A normal dog usually defecates one to four times each day. The consistency and quantity of faeces produced will depend on many factors – particularly the nature of his diet. A healthy dog fed on a good-quality diet should produce faeces that are well-formed and firm, not sloppy.

Causes

Diarrhoea may be a symptom of any disease that affects normal bowel movements, reduces the ability of the bowel wall to absorb fluid, or stimulates it to pour more fluid than normal into the digestive system. For instance, approximately 3 litres (5 pints) of fluid, made up of water ingested through drinking and with food, together with saliva and other secretions, may enter the digestive system of an average 20 kg (44 lb) springer spaniel every 24 hours. About 95 per cent of this fluid may be absorbed back into his body, and his faeces will contain 150 ml (¼ pt) of water. If his faeces were suddenly to contain just 20 ml (less than 1 fl oz) more water, he would have diarrhoea. Parts of the large bowel are also prone to inflammation: this is called colitis.

Underlying causes of diarrhoea include over-eating, diet changes, digestive-enzyme deficiencies, impaired digestion, damage to the intestinal wall by a foreign body (see pages 34–5), bacterial infections and viral infections such as canine parvovirus (see page 84).

Is it serious?

Diarrhoea should always be taken seriously. Most sudden episodes are mild and respond to symptomatic treatment, but some cases of acute diarrhoea – such as those caused by canine parvovirus (see page 84) – may be life-threatening. Managing longstanding diarrhoea can be very difficult, and the sooner such cases are investigated, the better.

Dogs at risk

All dogs are at risk, but puppies may be more prone to diarrhoea caused by dietary upsets, infections and parasitic intestinal worms (see pages 32–4). Exocrine pancreatic insufficiency, a digestive disorder, is especially common in German shepherd dogs. Older dogs are more likely to suffer from cancer affecting the digestive system.

Action

If your dog has mild diarrhoea, contact your vet centre for advice. You may need to arrange for him to be examined.

If your dog suffers a bout of severe diarrhoea, shows symptoms such as lethargy or vomiting, or is far from his normal self, contact your vet centre immediately.

If your dog suffers a bout of obvious diarrhoea but seems to be in all other respects his normal self, give him water only for 24 hours. If after this he still has diarrhoea, withhold his food for a further 24 hours. If the diarrhoea persists, or he begins to show other symptoms of being unwell, contact your vet.

If after 24 or 48 hours without food the symptoms have eased, you can offer your dog a small, highly digestible, low-fat, low-fibre meal of boiled rice, with a little hard-boiled egg, chicken or fish. Better still, offer a commercially prepared food for dogs with digestive disturbances (see page 104).

Continue to offer small meals every four hours during the day. If your dog stays well and his faeces firm up, gradually add his normal food, until he is back to his usual regime. If he has diarrhoea as soon as you feed him, contact your vet.

COMMON SYMPTOMS

The symptoms exhibited by a dog who is suffering from diarrhoea will depend on its cause and severity, but may include the following:
- Bulky faeces that are also softer in consistency than normal
- Large volumes of watery faeces that may be very dark in colour, foul-smelling and appear to contain blood.
- Colour changes to the faeces: some may be multi-coloured, ranging from brown and green to yellow.
- Greasy-looking faeces
- Pain on defecating

- Small amounts of faeces produced very frequently. An affected dog may strain to go to the toilet, and may have toileting 'accidents' indoors.
- A mixture of soft faeces and jelly-like mucus (this type of diarrhoea is typical in a case of colitis).
- Watery faeces mixed with jelly-like mucus and small amounts of blood.
- Obvious abdominal discomfort and general restlessness
- Gurgling bowel sounds
- Weight loss
- Vomiting (see pages 28–9)

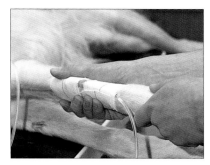

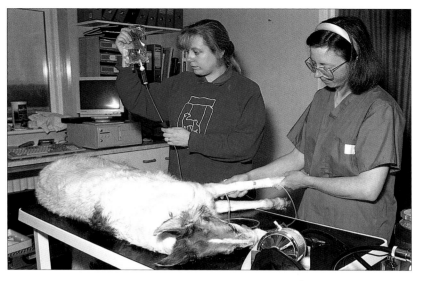

A dog with diarrhoea may soon become dehydrated. Administering fluids via an intravenous drip (above) can be a life-saving procedure.

The fluids enter the dog's circulation through a catheter, or fine tube, inserted into a vein – usually in a foreleg (right).

Your vet will examine your dog thoroughly and will consider his symptoms very carefully to try to identify the cause of the problem. Diagnosis can be very difficult, especially in longstanding cases, so he or she may carry out further investigations such as blood tests, analysis of your dog's faeces, X-ray and ultrasound investigations, examinations using an endoscope and microscopic examinations of small samples, or biopsies, of the bowel wall (see pages 91–3).

Your dog may need to stay at his vet centre for tests or for treatment, particularly if he is very unwell.

Treatment

The main aims are to give the dog's digestive system a rest, to replace lost body fluids and to deal with any identified cause. Many cases of diarrhoea can be managed with medicines alone, but others – such as intestinal obstructions due to foreign bodies (see pages 34–5) – may need surgery.

Cases of sudden and very severe diarrhoea need intensive therapy to control the symptoms and to treat the effects that repeated diarrhoea and fluid loss will have had on vital body chemistry. Treatment may include the following:
• No food given by mouth for 24 to 48 hours.
• Special fluids administered by mouth or directly into the blood via an intravenous drip (see page 95).
• Drugs given to control the dog's bowel movements.
• Anti-inflammatory medicines.
• Antibiotics, for instance where blood in the faeces suggests that the bowel wall is severely damaged.
• Wormers (see pages 32–4).
(Note: in most acute cases of severe diarrhoea, a basic treatment regime will be started while investigations are underway. If a specific cause is then identified, additional treatment may be implemented.)

Aftercare

At home, you must administer your dog's medicines (see pages 101–2) and carry out the specific dietary advice that you are given.

Avoid exercising your dog until he has completely recovered: your vet will advise you on this.

Prevention

It may be impossible to prevent many causes of diarrhoea, but the following are sensible precautions:
• Keep your dog's vaccinations fully up to date (see page 85).
• Discourage him from scavenging.
• Do not make sudden changes to his diet, or feed him your left-overs.
• Do not give him cows' milk, as many dogs are unable to produce enough of the enzyme needed to digest lactose in milk.
• If your dog has a large appetite, split his daily food allowance into two or more meals.
• Regularly treat your dog for intestinal worms (see pages 32–4).
• Feed him a high-quality commercially prepared food.

ZOONOSIS

Certain bacteria that may cause bouts of diarrhoea in dogs (such as salmonella and campylobacter) can also affect people. If your dog has diarrhoea, you and all your family should be extra-vigilant about your personal hygiene.

Parasitic intestinal-worm infestation

Parasites are organisms that live in or on other animals and derive their nourishment from them. There are a number of parasitic worms that may live and reproduce within a dog's intestines, but the specific worms that may affect your dog will depend on where you live and on his lifestyle. The two major types of worm to affect dogs are tapeworms and roundworms.

TAPEWORMS

There are a number of types of tapeworm that may affect dogs. Probably the most common type in the UK is *Dipylidium caninum*. These worms are flat, white and consist of many small segments; some may grow to 50 cm (20 in) in length.

Causes

Inside a dog's intestines, individual segments of an adult tapeworm, containing eggs, break off and then

pass to the outside world through the dog's anus. As these segments dry out they release their eggs. An immature flea (or a louse) in the environment may eat one or more of the eggs, which will continue to develop inside its body.

COMMON SYMPTOMS

Tapeworm infestations in dogs are often not noticed by the dogs' owners, but common symptoms include the following:
• Worm segments wriggling on the fur around the dog's anus, on his bedding or on the ground.
• The dog may 'scoot' his bottom along the ground, or lick and chew at his anus because of irritation.
• He may experience digestive disturbances such as diarrhoea (see pages 30–1), and general debility in a severe infestation.

As an adult, the flea will search for an animal to jump aboard in order to suck blood: this may be the same dog, another dog, a cat or even a person.

During its feeding activities the flea may create either mild or severe irritation (see page 56), causing the animal to nibble at and groom his skin. In doing so, he may swallow the flea. This will then be digested, releasing one or more immature tapeworms into the dog's intestines where they will develop into adults. And so the cycle continues.

Is it serious?

Dipylidium caninum rarely causes serious problems in adult dogs. However, as people can also be infested by this kind of tapeworm (see below), its existence should be taken seriously.

Dogs at risk

If there are fleas or lice in the environment that are carrying the immature tapeworms, all dogs – including young puppies – will be at risk of infestation.

Action

Assume that your dog is infested with tapeworms, and adopt a thorough prevention campaign (see opposite, above).

TAPEWORM INFESTATION

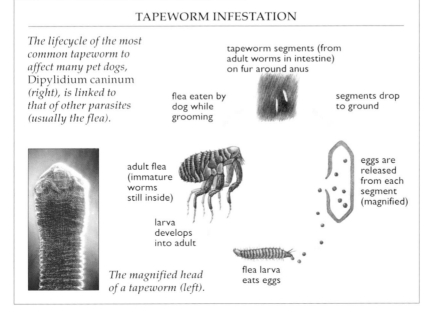

The lifecycle of the most common tapeworm to affect many pet dogs, Dipylidium caninum *(right), is linked to that of other parasites (usually the flea).*

tapeworm segments (from adult worms in intestine) on fur around anus

flea eaten by dog while grooming

segments drop to ground

adult flea (immature worms still inside)

eggs are released from each segment (magnified)

larva develops into adult

flea larva eats eggs

The magnified head of a tapeworm (left).

ZOONOSIS

Dipylidium caninum worms can affect people, but this only occurs very rarely. While playing with a dog, a person could swallow a flea containing a tapeworm egg. Once digested, the immature tapeworm would be able to develop into an adult in that person's intestines.

Worming a dog for tapeworms is easy and effective, so there will probably be little point in trying to prove whether your dog is infested with them before he is treated.

However, a veterinary nurse or your vet would be able to do so by looking for segments of tapeworm in a sample of your dog's faeces, using a microscope.

Prevention

Using a 'wormer' recommended by your vet centre, begin dosing your dog as soon as he comes to live with you, and keep doing so at regular intervals. I recommend my clients to treat their dogs for tapeworms every two to three months. Wormers are given by mouth (see pages 101–2), or by injection.

Part of your campaign against tapeworms should also include thorough and appropriate flea control, both on your dog and in your house (see page 59).

ROUNDWORMS

There are many different kinds of roundworm that may infest a dog's intestines, including hookworms and whipworms.

Perhaps the most prevalent roundworm in the UK is *Toxocara canis*, which has a complicated lifecycle that may involve other animals such as birds and rodents.

Some older dogs – particularly bitches after whelping – may have adult egg-laying roundworms in their intestines, but almost all puppies are infested at birth.

Causes

The most common way for a puppy to become infested is directly from his mother while he is still inside her uterus. Having been infested in this way, a puppy may have egg-laying adults inside him by the time he is three weeks old.

ROUNDWORM INFESTATION

The most important sources of Toxocara canis *roundworm infestation.*

foetus becomes infested before birth, in uterus

puppies become infested through drinking milk

puppy becomes infested by picking up and swallowing eggs in environment

In a severe infestation (left), adult roundworms may form knotted balls inside a puppy's intestines.

An egg-laying adult worm may produce several hundred thousand eggs a day, which pass out in the puppy's faeces. These eggs are very hardy and may survive for three years, but they cannot immediately infest another dog.

After two to three weeks in summer (longer in winter), eggs continue their development and may be swallowed by the same or another dog; they will hatch out in the intestines, and the immature worms will find their way into the blood. Some may pass through the liver and lungs, before being coughed up and swallowed back into the intestines to mature; others

---

COMMON SYMPTOMS

Most roundworm infestations in dogs of any age will pass unnoticed by the dogs' owners. However, in the worst infestations, any of the following symptoms may be apparent:
• Before he is 12 days old, an affected puppy may have noisy breathing and a nasal discharge due to the movement of immature roundworms through his respiratory system.

• In a two-week-old puppy the worms may cause vomiting, diarrhoea and stunted growth.
• A puppy of six to 12 weeks old who has not been wormed may suffer from severe vomiting and diarrhoea, and may be very pot-bellied.
• Dead and dying worms may be passed in a puppy's faeces, and will be easy to spot.

ZOONOSIS

Very rarely, people – particularly children – are affected by immature *Toxocara canis* roundworms, having accidentally ingested eggs. (It is very unlikely that a person would pick up eggs capable of infesting them by touching a dog, because the eggs take two to three weeks to reach that stage.) Inside a human's intestines the eggs will hatch, and immature worms may cause damage and disease as they move around the body (the worms will not develop into adults).

In order to reduce the chances of infestation, children must wash their hands before eating, food should be covered to prevent contamination by flies, and dog faeces should be cleared up immediately, before roundworm eggs are able to develop.

go to tissues such as the muscles, and then become dormant. (In young puppies, the majority take the route through the liver and lungs; in most older puppies and adult dogs they go to the tissues.)

Most adult dogs have dormant roundworms in certain tissues, but a remarkable thing happens in pregnant bitches. After about day 42 of pregnancy, some immature roundworms become active and enter the developing foetuses through their placentas. A bitch will also pass immature worms to her puppies via her milk.

Is it serious?

An infestation may cause serious digestive disturbances and even blockages, so *Toxocara* roundworms must be taken seriously.

Dogs at risk

All dogs are at risk, particularly unborn and very young puppies.

Action

It is fair to assume that all puppies will be born already infested with *Toxocara* roundworms, so you must adopt a prevention campaign using a 'wormer' recommended by your vet centre. The precise timing and method of treatment will depend on the age of your dog and on the product that you use (see below).

Your dog's faeces could be examined for roundworm eggs, but – as with tapeworms – worming is a simple and effective procedure, so this is not really necessary.

Prevention

All puppies should be treated with an effective wormer at appropriate intervals. A common regime is to worm puppies at two weeks old, then every two weeks until they are 12 weeks old. After this, most vets recommend worming every three months. Wormers are available as liquids, tablets or powders, and are given by mouth (see pages 101–2). Some products are effective against tapeworms and roundworms.

To reduce the contamination of the environment with roundworm eggs, clean up your dog's faeces as soon as possible. Remember that eggs may survive for three years, and are not killed by disinfectants.

Digestive-system foreign body

A foreign body is any object that is in an abnormal, unnatural or unusual place. In terms of a dog's digestive system, a foreign body is any solid object that is not considered a food item.

Typical examples of foreign bodies include paper, fragments of wood (swallowed when a dog chews sticks), stones, wrappers from food, pieces of bone, balls, corn cobs, string and fishing hooks.

Causes

Dogs are often indiscriminate about what they eat. New and interesting objects are frequently investigated by mouth, before being pulled to pieces. Faced with the decision of whether to spit out an object or to swallow it, many dogs will go for the gulp. As a result, they regularly ingest foreign bodies of all shapes, sizes and structures.

Some objects will be vomited back or may pass through a dog's digestive system with no problems. (Interestingly, foreign bodies are often discovered in dogs' stomachs when the dogs are X-rayed for other reasons. It seems that foreign bodies in the stomach are tolerated well, unless they block the entrance to the small intestine.)

COMMON SYMPTOMS

A foreign body may be a problem in the oesophagus, stomach or intestines. Symptoms will vary depending on the location of the object, the irritation it causes and the degree to which it blocks the digestive system, but may include:
• Excessive drooling (especially in an obstruction of the oesophagus)
• Regurgitation (perhaps for some weeks in a partial obstruction)
• Vomiting (see pages 28–9)
• Abdominal swelling
• Reluctance to eat and debility
• Constipation (see page 37)

Other foreign bodies – such as a fishing hook – may become impaled in the wall of the oesophagus, the stomach or the intestines. Large and irregularly shaped objects – such as pieces of bone or corn cobs – could also become stuck and block a dog's digestive system.

Is it serious?

Yes: a foreign body in the digestive system can be life-threatening.

Dogs at risk

All dogs are at risk of picking up a foreign body, but compulsive scavengers will be at greater risk.

Problems with foreign bodies in the oesophagus seem to be most common in the West Highland white and cairn terriers, and in the labrador retriever.

Action

If you think or know that your dog has swallowed a foreign body, or if he shows any of the symptoms described, contact your vet centre

A dog's natural instinct is to scavenge, although some dogs do so much more than others. Do not give your dog the opportunity to rifle through your refuse.

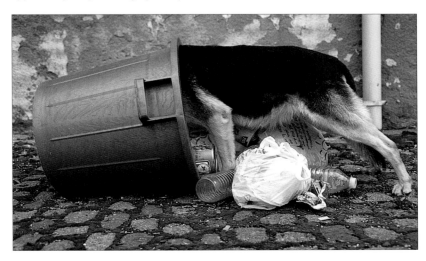

immediately. Do not allow your dog to take anything by mouth and do not exercise him until you have spoken to your vet.

Your vet will examine your dog thoroughly. Depending on the findings of this initial examination, he or she may carry out abdominal X-ray or ultrasound investigations (see page 92).

Treatment

Your vet may decide to observe your dog for a period, or to operate on him straight away. If your dog has been vomiting, he may be given fluids through an intravenous drip (see page 95), and he will almost certainly be treated with antibiotics.

Surgery • If the foreign body is stuck in your dog's oesophagus, surgery to remove it, using an endoscope (see page 91), may be carried out. If this procedure is unsuccessful, your dog may need open-chest surgery. If the foreign body is lodged in your dog's stomach or intestines, your vet may well open his abdomen to remove the object through the intestinal wall. If a piece of bowel has been damaged, your vet may need to remove it.

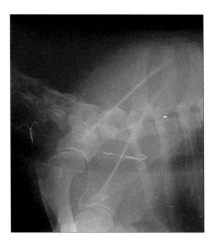

This X-ray of a dalmation reveals two fishing hooks stuck in his oesophagus. Others were found in his stomach, all attached to the same fishing line.

Aftercare

After surgery, your dog will have to stay in at your vet centre for at least one night for monitoring and drug administration. Your vet will only discharge him when he is well on the way to recovery.

At home, you must administer any prescribed drugs and follow the feeding advice that you are given. You must monitor your dog's food intake, as well as his general disposition and bowel movements, for discussion at his check-ups.

Prevention

Never leave your dog unsupervised with access to objects that he could swallow. Do not leave any rubbish or food waste within his reach, and remember that dogs are perfectly capable of opening kitchen bins.

Whenever possible, discourage your dog from scavenging by diverting his attention. Teach him the command to 'drop' so that, if you catch him with a potentially dangerous object in his mouth, he will spit rather than swallow.

Anal-sac disorders

The anal sacs are two pockets on either side of a dog's anal ring. Each is connected to the skin's surface by a single tube that opens close to the hairline around the anus. The sacs produce a light brown, oily liquid, some of which may be expressed when the dog produces faeces.

This oily liquid smells extremely unpleasant to us, but it may have an important role in social recognition between dogs. Two main conditions are associated with the anal sacs: overfilling and infection.

COMMON SYMPTOMS

Whether the anal sacs are overfull or infected, the early symptoms may include the following:
• Licking under the tail
• Chewing at one or more feet
• Chewing at the hindquarters and flanks, especially in dogs who for reasons such as obesity are unable to reach under their tails.
• An affected dog may 'scoot' his bottom along the ground.
• Distended anal sacs may cause obvious swellings.
• An infected anal sac that has abscessated may burst and then discharge its contents, including pus, blood and foul-smelling liquid.

The anal sacs lie under the skin and between the muscles that control a dog's anal sphincter.

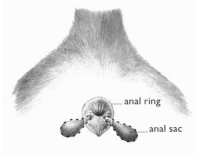

anal ring

anal sac

Causes

Overfilling may be caused by a change in consistency of the anal-sac liquid, making it difficult to express naturally, or by an increase in its production rate. A change in muscle tone around the anus may also affect the efficiency with which the sacs express their contents, as may an alteration in the form and the consistency of a dog's faeces.

Overfilling is often followed by infection, due to impaction and fermentation of the sac contents.

Is it serious?

Anal-sac impaction causes a dog obvious distress. An infection appears to be even more painful, and may turn into an abscess that eventually bursts. By attempting to empty and clean around infected anal sacs with his tongue, a dog may also develop pharyngitis and tonsillitis (see page 23).

Dogs at risk

An anal-sac disorder may affect any dog of any age or sex, but smaller breeds – such as the miniature and toy poodle – seem to suffer more than most. Dogs with other skin conditions, such as seborrhoea (see page 63), may be more at risk. Some dogs never suffer from anal-sac conditions, while many who do often have problems regularly.

Action

If your dog is showing any of the symptoms described, take him to your vet. If he is causing damage to his skin through licking or chewing at it, if he is distressed and cannot relax, or if an anal-sac abscess has burst, you should make this visit as soon as possible.

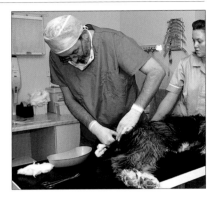

A dog who has severely impacted and infected anal sacs may need to be anaesthetized in order to be treated.

Your vet will carry out a rectal examination to determine whether your dog's anal sacs are full and/or impacted. By emptying a little fluid from them and inspecting its colour, he or she may be able to identify whether the sacs are infected.

Treatment

If your dog's anal sacs are overfull or impacted, your vet or a nurse will empty them. Your dog is unlikely to enjoy this any more than the person who inflicts it on him!

If the sacs are infected, your vet may wash them out under a general anaesthetic (see pages 96–7) before filling the sacs with antibiotic cream or ointment. Anti-inflammatory medicines may also be required.

For dogs who regularly suffer from overfull anal sacs, surgery to remove the sacs is an option.

Aftercare

At home, you must administer your dog's prescribed medicines. If he has had a burst anal-sac abscess, you will need to bathe and clean the wound with warm, salty water.

Constipation

A dog is constipated if he defecates less frequently than usual, or not at all. The number of times a day that a normal dog defecates will depend on his diet, and also on the personal peculiarities of his digestive system. Every dog is different, but most will defecate one to four times a day.

Causes

Constipation in dogs has a number of causes, including intestinal blockage by a foreign body (see pages 34–5) or a tumour, nerve damage, an enlarged prostate gland (see page 73), pain on defecation (in males), or any debilitating disease. Apparent constipation may occur due to a reduced appetite, or due to a lack of exercise in older dogs.

Is it serious?

Constipation is often the result of major underlying disease, so all cases should be taken seriously.

COMMON SYMPTOMS

- No faeces, or the production of less faeces than normal.
- The production of very dry and hard faeces.
- Straining and discomfort during attempts to defecate
- Restlessness
- General debility

Dogs at risk

All dogs are at risk of constipation.

Action

If your dog exhibits any of the symptoms described, contact your vet centre immediately.

To try to identify the cause of the constipation, your vet will carry out a physical and rectal examination. He or she may also undertake blood tests, X-rays and ultrasound investigations (see pages 92–3).

Treatment

Therapy for constipation involves relieving the symptoms, treating the cause (where possible) and instituting measures to prevent its recurrence (see below).

The symptomatic therapy may include laxatives, enemas to remove impacted faeces and fluids given via intravenous drip (see page 95).

Aftercare

Once your dog's bowels have been cleared you may need to carry out a number of measures, on your vet's advice, aimed at preventing the recurrence of the constipation.

Prevention

Preventive measures may include changing your dog's diet, adding laxatives and/or faecal softeners to his food and implementing a more regular exercise schedule.

Flatulence

Flatulence – often referred to as 'passing wind' – is the emission of gas from a dog's anus.

Causes

Gas may accumulate in a dog's intestines through swallowed air (usually due to gulping food or panting), through the diffusion of gas from his blood into his intestines, or through chemical reactions within the intestines. Fermentation of poorly digested food in the large intestine may also cause flatulence.

Is it serious?

Flatulence may be a symptom of other, more serious conditions affecting the digestive system.

Dogs at risk

Any dog may be flatulent, but those of the brachycephalic breeds – with their flat faces (see page 27) – may swallow more air than other dogs.

Action

You should discuss your dog's diet with your vet or a veterinary nurse.

COMMON SYMPTOMS

- An unpleasant odour in the local environment of an affected dog.
- A characteristic sound that tends to be peculiar to individual dogs.

Prevention

Control your dog's air-swallowing by feeding more, smaller meals. If he gulps his food, spread it thinly in a large, shallow bowl, or place a large, smooth stone in the bowl to make him eat more slowly. Feed him away from other dogs so that he feels less need to bolt his food.

Avoid using poorer-quality foods, those high in fibre, and those containing soya beans or wheat, and do not feed strong-flavoured, sulphur-containing vegetables, milk or high-protein foods if possible.

Avoid vitamin and mineral supplements, as these may promote fermentation in the large intestine.

Heart

Like a human, a dog only remains alive thanks to the unrelenting efforts of just one muscle: his heart. Unfortunately, a dog's heart is vulnerable to a number of specific conditions. Any of these may lead on to a syndrome called heart failure, in which the dog's circulatory system is unable to compensate for the effects of the underlying heart disease. This is a common dog health problem encountered by vets. Preventive measures against heartworm infestations (see pages 40–1) are essential in some countries.

Heart failure

Heart failure occurs when any kind of heart disease becomes so severe that a dog's heart is unable to circulate enough blood to meet all the needs of his body tissues. As a result of associated blood-pressure abnormalities, fluid may begin to pool in some of his tissues, and the blood supply decreases to those body tissues that are furthest away from the heart.

Causes

Any form of heart disease can cause this condition. A dog may be born with a defect that leads on to heart failure – such as a hole in the heart or a major blood vessel positioned wrongly – but in most cases heart failure is associated with an underlying heart disease that is not present at birth. These diseases include the following:
• Long-term disease of the major internal heart valves, making the valves ineffective as seals.
• Diseases of the heart muscle.
• An infestation of heartworms (see pages 40–1).
• Diseases of the tissues that surround the heart, leading to a build-up of fluid.
• Electrical disorders of the heart, affecting its beat rhythm and rate.
• Bacterial infections of the interior lining of the heart.
• Tumours of the heart.

Is it serious?

Heart failure is obviously a very serious, life-threatening condition.

Dogs at risk

Certain kinds of dog are prone to specific types of heart disease. For instance, heart-valve disorders are most common in middle-aged and older dogs, and in toy, miniature and small breeds, especially the Cavalier King Charles spaniel, chihuahua, cocker spaniel, poodle and Yorkshire terrier.

Heart-muscle disorders most commonly affect the boxer, cocker spaniel and doberman pinscher, as well as giant breeds, especially the Great Dane, Irish wolfhound, St Bernard and Newfoundland.

Action

Your dog should have a thorough examination by his vet at least once a year, even if he seems perfectly healthy. This will ensure that any of the earliest and most subtle symptoms of heart disease are identified. Your vet will then be able to monitor your dog's heart, and begin appropriate treatment.

If your dog is suffering from any of the symptoms described, take

---

COMMON SYMPTOMS

In the earliest stages of heart failure a dog may not show any symptoms, because changes that occur in his body will help to compensate for his failing heart. However, heart disease may still be detectable by a vet at an early stage (see right).

As the condition progresses, the dog will begin to exhibit symptoms. At first, this may only happen when his heart is under stress, such as on exercise, but later on his quality of life will deteriorate as he develops symptoms that are obvious on mild exercise or even at rest.

Typical symptoms are mainly due to the build-up of fluid in the lungs and/or abdomen, to an increase in the size of the heart as it tries to compensate for its own failure, and

to the inefficient pumping of blood around the body. They may include the following:
• Exhaustion on exercise
• Coughing
• An increased breathing rate
• Obvious distress when the dog is trying to breathe.
• Abdominal swelling
• Weakness and lethargy
• Cold extremities
• Pale gums
• Fainting
• Weight loss
• Reluctance to eat
• Depression
(Note: in some dogs, symptoms of heart failure develop quite gradually; in others, severe symptoms may appear to develop very suddenly.)

him to your vet as soon as possible. If he collapses or develops any other severe symptoms, such as breathing difficulties, contact your vet centre as an emergency, and carry out first aid until your vet takes over (see pages 116–17).

Your vet will take a detailed history of your dog's symptoms, and will then carry out specific investigations to confirm heart failure and to try to identify its cause. These may include any of the following procedures:

• Listening to your dog's chest with a stethoscope (see page 91) to identify symptoms such as a heart murmur that may indicate turbulent blood flow (for example, as a result of a leaking heart valve), heart-rate abnormalities, or fluid accumulation in the lungs.

• X-ray investigations to determine the size of the heart and the major blood vessels, and any changes affecting the lungs and airways.

• ECG, or electrocardiography, examinations (see page 92) to

THE ANATOMY OF A DOG'S HEART (SIDE VIEW)

A dog's heart lies almost upright in his chest. It is surrounded by the lungs, and is protected from injury by the rib cage.

lung
shoulder blade
rib
diaphragm
heart
sternum
(breast bone)

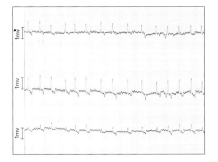

identify electrical disturbances in your dog's heart (he may be fitted with a mobile ECG recorder that will record his heart's electrical activity over a 24-hour period).

• Ultrasound investigations (see page 92).

• Blood tests (see page 93).

An ECG machine records the electrical activity of a dog's heart. The ECG trace below is from a labrador retriever with a healthy heart: notice the straight lines between the 'spike clumps'. The traces on the left are from a dog who has a condition called atrial fibrillation: this is characterized by erratic electrical activity in the heart, identified by the saw-shaped lines between the 'spike clumps'. These three traces were taken with the machine on different settings.

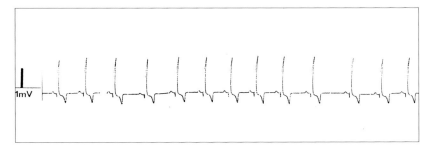

Treatment

The precise treatment will depend on the severity of your dog's heart condition, and on any underlying specific heart disease that your vet is able to identify.

The treatment of heart failure is aimed at controlling the symptoms. It is generally impossible to correct the cause of the condition, so the treatment will normally continue for the rest of the dog's life. Key features of treatment are as follows.

Exercise control • It is important that a dog who has heart failure does not over-exert himself. In a severe case, exercise control may include periods of bed-rest.

Dietary management • An obese dog will be put on a suitable weight-reduction programme (see pages 82–3). A low-salt diet is an important part of treatment in almost all cases, and specially formulated low-salt diets are available (see page 104).

Drugs • A whole range of drugs is used in the management of heart failure. Those that your vet uses will depend on the severity of your dog's condition, but

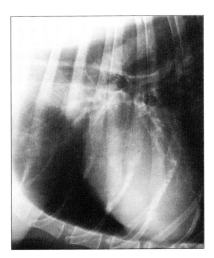

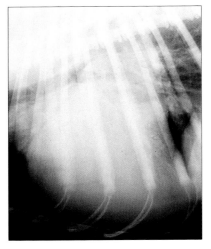

In the above X-ray of a healthy boxer's chest, the heart appears as a grey/white oval surrounded by the lungs (the black area). In the second X-ray, of a spaniel

with heart failure (caused by a heart-muscle condition), the heart is greatly enlarged; fluid has also accumulated in the lungs, around the base of the heart.

Pacemakers • In certain specific cases of electrical abnormalities in the heart, a pacemaker may be fitted to the dog to regulate his heart rhythm and rate.

If your dog is in advanced heart failure, he is likely to be kept in at your vet centre for intensive care that may include oxygen therapy, the administration of medicines by intravenous drip (see page 95) and the drainage of any life-threatening build-ups of fluid, as well as drug treatment. He will only be allowed home when his condition is stable.

Aftercare

You must administer your dog's medicines (see pages 101–2), adapt his diet if necessary and monitor his progress by weighing him, measuring his breathing rate and evaluating his response to exertion. He will need regular check-ups.

Prevention

Obesity is extremely likely to hasten the onset of severe heart failure in a dog with heart disease, and this is one very good reason why all dogs should be kept at their ideal weight (see pages 82–3).

commonly employed drugs include the following:
• Diuretics that help to remove unwanted fluid build-ups.
• Drugs that help to dilate blood vessels, and therefore reduce the workload on the failing heart.
• Drugs that control the beat rhythm and rate of the heart.

• Drugs that increase the strength of heart contractions.
• Drugs that help to open up the airways, and so make it easier for an affected dog to breathe.
Surgery • Certain anatomical defects affecting a dog's heart, that are present at birth, may be correctable by surgery.

Heartworm infestation

This heart condition involves an infestation with parasitic worms, which cause disease by damaging the lining of the heart and its major blood vessels. Historically, heartworm infestation appears to have been limited to dogs living in tropical and subtropical parts of the world, but it is now also being diagnosed in cooler regions.

Causes

Adult heartworms grow to a length of up to 25 cm (10 in) inside the heart and main blood vessels that

lead to the lungs. Females produce immature worms, or microfilariae, that circulate in a dog's blood for as long as two years and may be picked up in blood sucked by a mosquito. Inside the mosquito's body they develop into larvae that will be injected into another dog when the mosquito feeds again.

About six months after being injected into an uninfested dog, the larvae will have grown into adult worms and produced their own offspring. These will cruise the blood vessels of this now-infested

dog, waiting to be picked up by another mosquito.

Is it serious?

Heartworms can cause serious, life-threatening disease. Treatment of an established infestation of these worms in a dog can also be very hazardous (see opposite).

Dogs at risk

All dogs, but particularly those living outdoors in mosquito-ridden environments, are at risk of picking up a heartworm infestation.

Action

You must not wait for your dog to become infested with heartworms before taking action. If you live in a region in which heartworms are known to be a problem (ask at your vet centre for advice on the situation in your area), you should medicate your dog on a routine basis in order to prevent him from becoming infested (see below).

If your dog exhibits any of the symptoms typical of a heartworm infestation, your vet will examine him thoroughly before carrying out further investigations. These may include blood and urine tests, X-ray and ultrasound investigations of his chest and ECG examinations (see pages 92–3).

Treatment

Treatment of an infested dog is both complicated and potentially hazardous. The specific treatment regime that is used will depend on the severity of the symptoms and the level of your dog's heartworm burden, but will generally involve the following three phases:

Symptomatic treatment • This will be implemented first. The

HEARTWORM INFESTATION

The lifecycle of the canine heartworm, Dirofilaria immitis, *relies on mosquitoes to transfer infestation from one dog to another.*

Between two and four months after being injected into a healthy dog, developing heartworms will be found inside his heart. It will take a further two months for them to mature and produce their own microfilariae.

An infested dog has immature worms – called microfilariae – in his blood. By feeding on this blood a mosquito picks up worms, which develop into larvae in the mosquito's body.

By biting through an uninfested dog's skin to suck another blood meal, the contaminated mosquito injects heartworm larvae into its victim.

COMMON SYMPTOMS

A dog with a heartworm burden will exhibit symptoms of heart failure (see page 38). Symptoms may take three years to develop after the initial infestation, and may include the following:
• Exhaustion on normal exercise
• Coughing
• Breathing difficulties
• Weakness
• A dog with a severe infestation may also develop symptoms associated with kidney and liver disorders (see pages 67 and 78).

---

purpose of this treatment is to ensure that your dog will be as fit and healthy as possible before any toxic drugs are administered to kill the heartworms.

Toxic-drug treatment • In this second stage of treatment, drugs will be given to eliminate the adult heartworms. Your dog will need to be kept in at his vet centre during this treatment, so that he can be bed-rested and monitored for signs of illness that may be associated with the administration of these drugs.

Further drug treatment • This will be used to eliminate the microfilariae that are circulating in your dog's bloodstream.

Prevention

Heartworm infestations in dogs can be prevented by the routine administration of drugs to kill the larvae. You should discuss with your vet or a veterinary nurse

the drug options that are currently available in your area or country. Preventive treatment should begin one to two months in advance of the mosquito season, and should be continued for one full month after the season has ended.

Prior to beginning treatment, your vet will carry out a blood test to confirm that your dog is not already infested with heartworms. In addition, it is likely that he or she will wish to monitor your dog's heartworm status by carrying out a similar blood test every year.

If you live in a mosquito-ridden area in which heartworms in dogs are known to be a problem, or if you are moving to such an area with your dog, you should ask at your vet centre for advice on creating a heartworm-prevention programme for him. This should be incorporated into his overall preventive-healthcare plan (see pages 112–13).

Airways

Adog's airways consist of his nasal cavities, his windpipe and the network of smaller pipes that connect this to microscopic chambers in the lungs where the exchange of oxygen and carbon dioxide to and from the blood takes place. The sensitive lining of a dog's airways is vulnerable to attack by infectious organisms, and also to chronic inflammatory damage. If you take your dog to places where many other dogs congregate – such as boarding kennels – he will be at risk of catching contagious respiratory disease.

Contagious respiratory disease

This is a common, often multiple infection of a dog's windpipe and smaller airways. It is very easily transmitted between dogs, and is known as 'kennel cough'.

Causes

The organisms that are commonly associated with this condition are a bacterium called *Bordetella bronchiseptica*, a virus called canine adenovirus 2 (CAV-2) and a virus called canine parainfluenza virus. The presence of these organisms in the airways causes inflammation of the lining tissues. Any of the above organisms may be the sole cause of contagious respiratory disease, or more than one organism may be involved at a time.

Is it serious?

In almost all cases, contagious respiratory disease is not serious. Most infected dogs recover within 10 days, even without treatment.

Dogs at risk

All dogs entering an environment in which dogs are kept in groups – particularly where the population of dogs is constantly changing, such as in kennels – are at risk.

Action

If your dog develops a 'honking' cough within a few days of being exposed to a dog with contagious respiratory disease, or to a group of unknown dogs (for instance, in kennels), he may have picked up an infection. Gently pull on his collar: if he immediately coughs, his windpipe may be inflamed.

If your dog is otherwise well, let the condition take its course but keep him isolated from any other dogs. However, if he coughs so much that he

The Bordetella *vaccine (in the UK) is sprayed up a dog's nose. It should be given four weeks before the dog enters a high-risk area, such as kennels.*

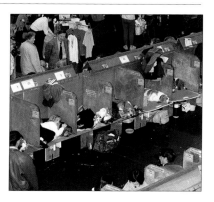

Dog shows and boarding kennels are places in which contagious respiratory disease can quickly spread.

COMMON SYMPTOMS

Symptoms may appear in a healthy dog within five to 10 days of his contact with an infected dog. The symptoms may last just for a few days or linger for several weeks, and may include the following:
• A 'honking' cough that is usually worse on exercise or when the dog pulls against his lead.
• Productive coughing (in some, but not all cases).
• Frequent bouts of coughing, often ending in gagging or retching.
• A nasal discharge (in some cases)
• Most dogs remain fairly well in themselves, but some dogs may develop a fever and depression associated with a more serious infection of the lungs.

becomes distressed, if he develops other symptoms such as lethargy or reluctance to eat, or if his cough does not settle down within a week, take him to your vet.

Your vet will probably be able to confirm contagious respiratory disease by examining your dog, but will be unable to tell which organisms are involved without investigation. This may involve blood tests, as well as analysis of swabs taken from your dog's nose or pharynx and of mucus from his windpipe (see page 93).

If your dog is very unwell, your vet may also wish to carry out an X-ray investigation of his chest; this will be in order to look for any signs of associated lung damage.

Treatment
Depending on the severity of the condition, no treatment may be required, or your vet may prescribe antibiotics that you will need to administer to your dog at home (see pages 101–2).

Cough suppressants are now thought to be of little benefit.

Prevention
Vaccinations against all three of the main organisms involved in contagious respiratory disease are available. The vaccine against the CAV-2 virus is likely to be part of your dog's routine vaccinations; a parainfluenza virus vaccination may also be given (see page 85).

Discuss temporary vaccination against *Bordetella* bacteria with your vet before your dog enters a high-risk area; this may need to be repeated every six months.

Chronic bronchial disease

This disease actually covers a group of conditions that includes chronic bronchitis. They all cause increased resistance to the flow of air in, and particularly out, of a dog's lungs, and an overall reduction in his ability to breathe effectively.

Whatever its cause, the result of this condition is the same. The lining of the airways in the lungs becomes inflamed, and responds by producing more protective mucus than normal. The smaller airways become narrowed and, in time, recurrent inflammation causes permanent damage.

Causes
Chronic bronchial disease is much better understood in humans, in whom this disease may be due to long-term exposure to pollution, including cigarette smoke. As dogs share our air, they may be similarly affected. Obesity (see pages 82–3) may also be a contributing cause.

Is it serious?
The damage to the airways of a dog with this disease may be irreversible. The severe symptoms are extremely debilitating.

Dogs at risk
Due to the long-term nature of chronic bronchial disease, affected dogs are normally middle-aged or old. Small breeds seem especially prone, while overweight dogs suffer more severe symptoms.

Action
If your dog has a persistent cough or shows other symptoms listed below, take him to your vet. Do not ignore the symptoms, even if mild.

Your vet will examine your dog, and will then make further specific investigations. These may include blood tests, chest X-rays, analysis of mucus from his airways (see

COMMON SYMPTOMS
Typical symptoms are as follows (in some cases these may be mild, but in others they may be very severe and debilitating):
• Persistent coughing, continuing for several months
• Mucus may be coughed up
• Increased breathing rate
• Exhaustion on normal exercise

pages 92–3), and analysis of faeces to check for airway parasites.

Treatment
Your vet will prescribe medicines to reduce mucus production and inflammation of the airways, to control any bacterial infections and to open up the airways. If your dog is not coughing up mucus, cough suppressants may help, but are often thought to be of little benefit.

In many cases long-term therapy is required. Your vet may need to try various drugs before settling on the best combination for your dog.

Aftercare
Avoid exposing your dog to dry, dusty or polluted air: if you smoke, this is your excuse to stop! Cold air may also irritate his airways. Steam inhalation will relieve congestion, so keep your dog in the bathroom when you have a bath or a shower. Chest massage will also help: your vet will show you what to do.

Prevention
Try to keep your dog in a clean-air environment, and keep him at his ideal weight (see pages 82–3).

Joints, bones and ligaments

Most dogs – particularly large, athletic types – are active animals whose joints, bones and ligaments suffer from wear and tear in everyday life. Perhaps the most dramatic of injuries suffered by dogs are bone fractures, but modern orthopaedic-surgery techniques mean that the vast majority of fractures are now very treatable. Arthritis, on the other hand, is an extremely debilitating condition that is impossible to cure and, in many cases, difficult to control. Any lameness in a dog should never be dismissed, no matter how mild.

Lameness

A dog is described as lame if he appears to be unable to move or to bear weight on a leg normally.

Causes

Rather than being a condition in its own right, lameness is really a symptom of other underlying conditions, most of them painful.

These conditions may affect the feet, including the presence of foreign bodies – such as thorns or grass seeds – in the foot pads, cuts or other wounds, interdigital pyoderma (see page 62) or other painful skin conditions of the feet, or a broken claw (see page 65).

Other common causes include arthritis (see pages 46–7), bone fractures (see pages 48–9) and rupture of the cranial cruciate ligament in the knee (see page 53).

Action

If your dog is suddenly very lame and will not bear any weight on a leg, keep him rested and contact your vet centre as soon as possible.

Once you have identified the leg on which your dog is lame, manipulate every part of it gently. If you identify a spot that is obviously painful to your dog, examine that area in detail.

COMMON SYMPTOMS

- Reluctance to bear any weight on the affected leg.
- Scuffed claws or a broken claw on the foot of the affected leg.
- A hobbling gait
- An abnormal appearance to the affected leg.

If your dog is suffering from a milder degree of lameness, you should first try to identify which leg or legs are causing problems (in most cases of sudden lameness, only one leg is affected). If this is not immediately obvious, ask an assistant to walk and then trot your dog up and down on a hard surface, and watch the way he moves very carefully. A subtle lameness involving one of the forelegs will be easiest to pinpoint if you try to spot which of your dog's forelegs he lunges on to – and therefore is trying to take more weight on – when he is moving. This will be his good leg. (It is often easier to identify this lungeing movement when a dog is trotting along rather than walking.)

Once you have identified the leg that is causing the problem, examine every part of it

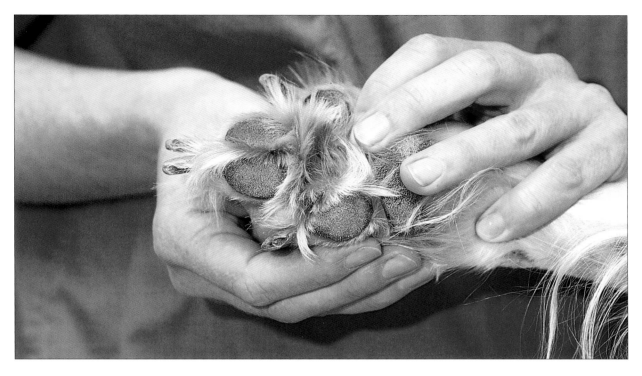

Sudden-onset, mild lameness is often due to a problem with the paw, such as a thorn stuck in a pad, grass seeds in the hair between the toes, or a damaged claw. Examine your dog's feet as part of routine health-checks (see pages 8–9).

thoroughly and systematically, beginning with each claw in turn. In case your dog should react aggressively due to any pain or discomfort that you may inflict, you should put a muzzle on him before you begin (see pages 98–9).

You should know when you locate a painful area by your dog's reaction to your manipulation of it. If you suspect that his response to being touched in a particular place may simply be due to his being ticklish or sensitive, examine the same area on the other leg and see how he responds.

Examine any painful area in greater detail: a magnifying glass may be helpful. If you discover a foreign body, such as a thorn, try to remove it (see below). If you

find a cut or other wound, deal with it in the appropriate manner (see pages 108–9). If you identify a painful joint that appears swollen, apply a cold compress, such as a cloth wetted with very cold water, or a bag of frozen peas.

If you cannot identify why your dog is lame, or the lameness is not completely resolved after 24 hours' rest, contact your vet centre.

Your vet will examine your dog to identify the lame leg (or legs), and will then check it in detail, to confirm your observations. In order to make an accurate diagnosis, he or she may also carry out further tests including joint manipulations, X-ray investigations (see page 92) and nerve tests, if appropriate.

Treatment

The precise treatment given in any case will depend on the underlying cause of the lameness.

REMOVING A FOREIGN BODY FROM YOUR DOG'S PAW

First muzzle your dog and ask an assistant to restrain him properly (see pages 98–9), then gently try to extract the foreign body using a pair of tweezers. If you manage to do so, bathe the affected paw in warm, salty water for a few minutes, and then bathe it with a veterinary antiseptic solution, before drying it off gently.

Keep a close eye on your dog's paw for several days. If it begins to swell, if your dog constantly tries to chew at it, or if he remains lame, contact your vet centre.

Arthritis

Dogs can suffer from different kinds of arthritis. The name literally means joint inflammation, but arthritis is much more complex than simple inflammation, so this can be rather misleading.

For instance, osteoarthritis is associated with the growth of new bone around a moveable joint, and with deterioration of the smooth cartilage that covers and protects the ends of the bones within it; the tissues that line the joint may not necessarily be inflamed.

Causes

The two forms of arthritis that are most commonly suffered by dogs are called traumatic arthritis and osteoarthritis. Traumatic arthritis is caused by sudden injury to a joint:

for example, as the result of a knock or sprain. The injury may include tearing or stretching of the soft tissues and ligaments within and surrounding the joint, and damage to the bones or their cartilage coverings within the joint.

Osteoarthritis may occur as a spontaneous condition, or may follow on from other kinds of joint abnormality. These may include hip dysplasia (see pages 50–1), osteochondritis dissecans, or OCD (a cartilage disease that commonly affects specific joints of certain breeds, such as the elbow in the labrador retriever and rottweiler), and joint dislocations that may make a joint unstable and therefore more susceptible to excessive and abnormal wear and tear.

Is it serious?

Traumatic arthritis in a dog's joint, resulting from a minor sprain, is very likely to be painful for a short while but not serious. However, the damage inflicted to a joint in, for instance, an impact with a car in a road-traffic accident may be much more serious and may also involve bone fractures within the joint that require surgery (see pages 48–9).

The seriousness of osteoarthritis will depend on the nature of any underlying cause, on the number and location of joints affected, and on the personality and health of the dog. An overweight dog will always suffer more than one of the correct weight. Some dogs – particularly most labrador retrievers,

A simple 'mattress' made from newspaper balls placed under a man-made fleece rug will be appreciated by a dog in pain.

COMMON SYMPTOMS

TRAUMATIC ARTHRITIS
- A swollen joint
- A painful joint, causing lameness on that leg (see pages 44–5) and resentment of the joint being manipulated in any way.

OSTEOARTHRITIS
- Lameness or stiffness: this may be mild or intermittent initially, but will gradually become worse over time.
- Typically, lameness or stiffness may be worse after the dog has been resting, and usually appears to wear off within a few minutes of his moving around.

in my experience – cope much better with pain and discomfort than others. However, arthritis should always be taken seriously.

Osteoarthritis is a progressive disease, and in some older animals may cause such severe disability that an arthritic dog's quality of life may be adversely affected.

Dogs at risk

Traumatic arthritis is perhaps most common in dogs who lead very athletic lives. Osteoarthritis is a recognized problem in breeds known to suffer from underlying causes, such as hip dysplasia (see pages 50–1). The development of osteoarthritis for unknown reasons seems more common in the chow chow, dalmatian and samoyed, as well as in retrievers and spaniels, but all dogs are vulnerable.

Action

If your dog suddenly begins to limp, treat him as described for lameness (see page 44).

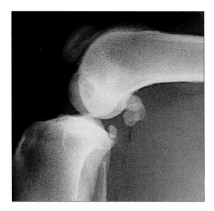

This is an X-ray picture of a stifle, or knee, joint in a normal dog; compare this with the very different X-ray picture on the right.

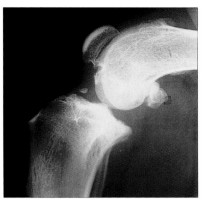

This X-ray shows changes associated with osteoarthritis: note the roughened bone edges. Use the drawing (right) to identify the features of this picture.

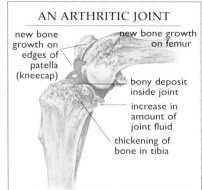

AN ARTHRITIC JOINT
new bone growth on edges of patella (kneecap)
new bone growth on femur
bony deposit inside joint
increase in amount of joint fluid
thickening of bone in tibia

A striking feature of a joint affected by osteoarthritis is the appearance of bony outgrowths, laid down in an attempt by the body to stabilize the damaged joint.

Even if your dog only limps occasionally, or is just a little stiff after rest, take him to see your vet. Do not wait until he is hobbling about: if he has osteoarthritis, the sooner you know, the sooner you can adopt measures that may slow the rate at which his condition will deteriorate. It will help your vet if you make notes on the nature and extent of your dog's symptoms.

When a dog becomes lame, many owners find it difficult to establish which leg is the painful one. With lameness affecting one or both hindlegs, this can be very tricky; foreleg lameness is much easier to identify (see page 44).

Your vet will consider the history of your dog's symptoms and will examine him at rest and, if it is appropriate, on exercise. You may be asked to trot your dog up and down on a flat surface a few times. The vet will also manipulate his joints in order to find out whether they are painful or stiff.

Once your vet has identified which joint or joints are affected, he or she may wish to carry out further investigations, including taking X-ray pictures and possibly analysing fluid samples taken from a swollen joint or joints.

Treatment

This will depend on the cause and on the severity of the arthritis. In an acute case, it is likely to include a short course of anti-inflammatory painkillers and strict rest. In a case of established osteoarthritis, it may include any of the following:

Medicines • Anti-inflammatory, painkilling medicines may be administered as a short course. If your vet prescribes these, do not think of them as miracle cures simply because your dog's stiffness disappears when he is on them. In most cases they are acting as painkillers, and will be less important in the long term than weight control and exercise management.

Exercise management • Carefully controlled exercise, with rest during painful episodes, should be implemented: follow your vet's advice. Regular short walks will help to maintain muscle bulk and prevent stiffness; too much or intermittent excessive exercise will aggravate arthritis. Your vet may also advise you to encourage your dog to swim.

Massage • Massaging your dog's joints, and physiotherapy, may be appropriate: ask your vet or a veterinary nurse for advice on the techniques to use.

Surgery • A dog who has severe osteoarthritis associated with hip dysplasia (see pages 50–1) may benefit from a hip-joint replacement. Surgery may also be needed in a case of traumatic arthritis, to repair severe joint damage such as a bone fracture or a torn ligament (see page 53).

Osteoarthritis is a progressive condition, so treatment will need to be adapted from time to time. Weight control (see pages 82–3) is perhaps the single most important feature of treatment for arthritis.

Prevention

Prompt medical treatment for any sprains, lifelong weight control, and responsible breeding to help to control hereditary joint disorders are important preventive measures.

Bone fracture

A bone is described as fractured when it has cracked, split, bent, shattered or snapped into two or more pieces. A so-called simple, or closed, fracture is one in which the overlying skin remains intact. In a compound, or open, fracture, there will be a hole through the skin, in the form of a wound, that leads down to where the bone (or bones) is damaged.

Although the bones of the legs and feet are perhaps those most commonly affected, any of a dog's bones may be fractured, including those of the skull, jaw, rib cage, spine, shoulder blades and pelvis.

Causes

Most fractures are caused by direct injury to bones, as a result of road-traffic accidents or falls. Other possible causes of fractures include being trodden on or kicked by another animal, excessive muscle contractions and gunshot injuries. Even everyday movements may be sufficient to fracture bones that are weakened by other conditions such as cancer (see pages 74–5).

Is it serious?

Bone, or orthopaedic, surgery for dogs is now very advanced (see opposite). It is possible to repair most fractures through surgery, although an affected dog may be permanently disabled to some extent if his injuries are severe.

Dogs at risk

All dogs are at risk of fracturing a bone, especially those dogs who stray near roads or who lead very athletic lives. Dogs with weak bones, such as very young puppies or those suffering from diseases affecting the bones – such as cancer (see pages 74–5) – may be more at risk of fracturing a bone than healthy adult dogs.

Action

If you know that your dog has been involved in an accident of any kind, you should take him for a check-up with your vet as soon as you can, even if he does not seem to be seriously injured.

Any of the symptoms associated with a bone fracture should be dealt with as emergencies until proven otherwise by your vet.

Following an accident, you may need to carry out appropriate first aid on your dog (see pages 116–17).

COMMON SYMPTOMS

These will depend on the bone or bones that are affected and on the type of fracture or fractures involved, but are likely to include the following:
• An obvious skin wound (the broken bone ends may be visible).
• Marked swelling of the tissues surrounding the fracture.
• Unusual behaviour resulting from pain, such as whining or aggression, especially when the dog is handled.
• An abnormal appearance or outline associated with the affected body part.
• Inability to use the affected body part. For instance, a broken leg will be held off the ground without bearing any weight, a major fracture of the spine or pelvis may cause paralysis and a fractured jaw may hang open.

COMMON TYPES OF BONE FRACTURE

Bone fractures are classified in the following ways: in a simple (closed) fracture the skin over the fracture is still intact; in a compound (open) fracture the skin and tissue over the pieces of bone are damaged and the bone is exposed. Whether closed or open, in a complete fracture the bone has separated into one or more parts, while a fracture that includes several bone fragments is described as comminuted.

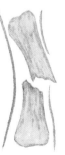

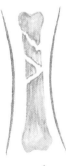

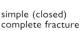
simple (closed) complete fracture

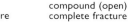
compound (open) complete fracture

simple (closed) complete comminuted fracture

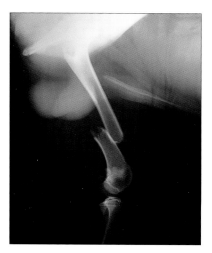

This is an X-ray picture of a simple (closed) complete fracture of the femur, or thigh bone, of a male dog.

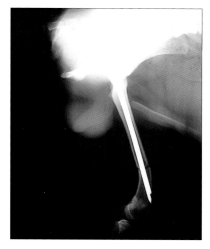

This picture shows the newly repaired fracture, with metal pins inserted into the marrow cavity of the broken bone.

Your vet will confirm a bone fracture by carrying out a thorough physical examination and taking X-ray pictures (see page 92).

In many cases, bone fractures are not the most serious of the injuries faced by a dog who has been involved in a major accident. If your dog is suffering from severe multiple injuries – perhaps as the result of a road-traffic accident – your vet will initially concentrate on keeping him alive. For this reason, he or she may only carry out immediate repairs to any fractures that are considered to be life-threatening, and may simply stabilize any less serious fractures on a temporary basis using splints or other dressings.

Your vet should administer painkillers to your dog, and may also treat him with antibiotics if this is necessary.

Treatment

A fractured bone will repair itself, provided that the broken ends are held in the correct positions to allow natural healing to take place. The aim of any fracture treatment is to put the broken pieces back into their normal anatomical relationship, and then to prevent them from moving as they heal.

The following are all commonly employed techniques (the one that is used will depend on the type of fracture and on its location):

Casts and splints • The broken bone ends will be manipulated back into their correct, normal alignment, and a rigid cast or splint will then be applied. Casts and splints may also be applied following other types of fracture repair, in order to provide extra support.

Insertion of a metal pin • In this surgical procedure, a pin (or pins) is inserted into the marrow cavity of a broken bone, to hold the two largest pieces in their normal position. Wires may then be tightened around the bones to help to prevent movement during healing, and to attach any smaller bone fragments.

Screws • Bone fragments may be repositioned using special metal screws.

Metal plates • These may be screwed on to two or more pieces of broken bone to hold them together.

External 'scaffolding' • Bone fragments in a leg fracture may be held rigidly in position by passing fine pins into the bones through the skin. In this type of repair, many pins are inserted and then bolted together on the outside of the leg to make a strong, supportive 'scaffold'.

The speed at which a fractured bone heals will depend on the age of the dog (in a puppy, a broken bone may be back to normal in six weeks; in an older dog, this may take four months), and on how closely together and how rigidly fixed the bone edges are during healing. Bones that have broken into just two pieces will generally heal faster than those broken into many fragments. The presence of infection will delay healing.

Your dog may stay in at your vet centre for the day of his operation, or for several days or even weeks.

Aftercare

At home, you must administer any prescribed medicines, such as painkillers, and keep dressings – including casts – clean and dry (see pages 108–9). Your vet will advise you as to the amount and type of movement that your dog can do.

Your vet will wish to see your dog for regular check-ups, and will take further X-ray pictures to see how the fracture is healing.

Any internal metalwork used to repair a fracture is likely to be left permanently in place, but your vet may remove any pins, screws, plates or wires if they could cause your dog further problems.

Hip dysplasia

A normal dog's hip joint comprises a ball-shaped piece of bone on the end of the femur, or thigh bone, which fits snugly into a smooth, deep, bony socket in the pelvis. Hip dysplasia is a very common condition, in which the hip joint is abnormally formed and the ball fits only loosely into its socket.

An affected hip joint suffers from abnormal and excessive wear and tear that commonly leads to osteoarthritis (see pages 46–7). This condition generally affects both of a dog's hip joints.

Causes

The development of hip dysplasia may depend on a dog's genetic make-up: this is a hereditary condition, and can be passed on from one generation to the next.

A dog's diet and exercise during his puppyhood are also relevant. Any feeding regime that promotes unnaturally rapid growth, and/or excessive exercise within the first year of life, may adversely affect the development of the hip joints.

Is it serious?

Hip dysplasia in dogs is a serious condition. It may not produce symptoms in all affected puppies, and nearly eight out of 10 of those who do suffer from symptoms show an improvement by the time they are about 15 months old and have stopped growing. However, the condition will often result in debilitating osteoarthritis of the hips as a dog grows older.

The individuals who are worst affected may be literally crippled by this condition when they are only a few years old.

Dogs at risk

As a general rule, hip dysplasia is common in most large breeds of dog, excepting the greyhound. Of the breeds surveyed by the current hip-dysplasia-control scheme in the UK, the following were considered some of the worst affected breeds:
• Airedale and Tibetan terriers
• Briard
• Brittany
• Bull mastiff

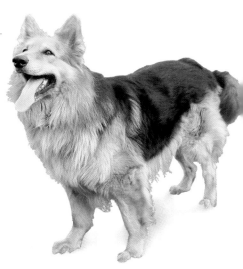

In the UK, the German shepherd is one of the dog breeds that is worst affected by hip dysplasia.

• Clumber, Sussex, Welsh springer and Irish water spaniels.
• English and Gordon setters
• German shepherd
• Golden retriever
• Hungarian puli
• Newfoundland
• Otterhound
• Shetland, Polish lowland and old English sheepdogs.
• St Bernard

Action

Whether you have a puppy or an older dog, if you are concerned about his gait or if he exhibits any of the other symptoms of hip dysplasia, contact your vet centre.

Your vet should examine your dog at rest and when moving. By manipulating his hip joints, he or she should be able to determine whether one or both is painful.

It can be difficult to examine a dog's hips properly when he is conscious, as he is likely to tense his muscles and to resist any manipulation of a painful joint

COMMON SYMPTOMS

The symptoms shown by a dog with hip dysplasia will depend on many factors, including the severity of the abnormality and his weight, lifestyle and age. Some puppies may suffer hip pain, typically at four to eight months old, but others may show no obvious symptoms, or simply an unusual gait. Sooner or later, most dogs with hip dysplasia develop osteoarthritis in their hips and will show symptoms associated with this painful condition (see pages 46–7). Typical symptoms of hip dysplasia may include:

• A swaying gait (most obvious from behind while a dog is walking).
• A 'bunny-hopping' gait, in which an affected dog uses both hindlegs together in order to bounce himself along (doing this reduces movement in the hip joints, and shifts more weight on to the forelegs).
• Limping on one hindleg only
• Apparent fatigue shown during normal exercise.
• Reluctance to stand
• Difficulty in climbing stairs
• Stiffness on rising after rest

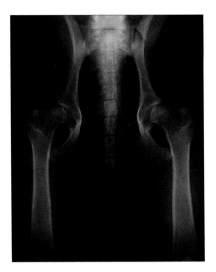

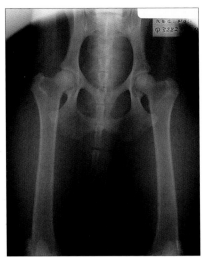

This dog's joints (above) are badly affected by hip dysplasia. The 'ball' at the end of each femur, or thigh bone, *is angular and does not fit snugly into its 'socket' in the pelvis. The second picture shows a normal pair of hips.*

or joints, so your vet may need to anaesthetize him in order to carry this out (see pages 96–7).

At the same time, he or she is likely to take an X-ray picture of the hips (see page 92), in order to confirm the nature and extent of any physical abnormalities in the hip joint or joints.

Treatment

Treatment for a puppy with known hip dysplasia is likely to include the following:

Exercise control • He should be exercised enough to promote development of strong muscles and supporting tissues around the hip joints, but excessive exercise must be avoided until he has reached maturity. About 10 minutes of lead walking four times a day is a regime that generally works well.

Dietary control • Overfeeding and excessive supplementation of the puppy's diet with vitamins and minerals should be stopped.

Painkillers • If a puppy is in pain despite appropriate changes to his exercise and diet regime, painkillers will make him feel more comfortable and therefore keener to take exercise, which will help to prevent joint stiffness and muscle wastage.

When fully grown, some affected dogs may benefit from surgery:

techniques include operations on two muscles situated close to the hip joints, reconstructive surgery of the pelvis, and even hip-joint replacement(s) in the worst cases.

A dog who goes on to suffer from osteoarthritis will be treated accordingly (see page 47).

Aftercare

At home, you must administer any prescribed medicines to your dog (see pages 101–2), and follow the exercise and diet regime that is recommended by your vet. You will need to take your dog back to your vet for regular check-ups.

Prevention

The development of all puppies should be carefully monitored by regular veterinary examinations and weighing, in order to make sure that they are not growing too quickly (see page 112). Puppies should also be exercised sensibly until they are fully grown.

The way in which hip dysplasia is passed from one generation to the next is not fully understood, but it is considered unwise and irresponsible to breed from badly affected dogs (see below).

HIP EXAMINATIONS

In order to help control hip dysplasia (in the UK), the British Veterinary Association and the Kennel Club run an X-ray-examination scheme, the purpose of which is to identify individuals who are most severely affected by the condition.

Hip X-rays taken when a dog is at least 12 months old are examined by a panel of orthopaedic experts, who award each dog a score of between 0 and 53 for each hip (the higher the score, the worse the hip dysplasia). The panel then calculates an average

combined score for both hips, and recommends that only dogs with a score of well below average for their breed should be used for breeding.

Before adopting a pure-bred puppy, make sure that his parents have been tested if they belong to a breed that is covered by the scheme. The staff at your vet centre will be able to advise you further.

If you live outside the UK, ask at your vet centre for details of any similar schemes that may currently be in operation in your country.

Intervertebral-disc protrusion

Between the bones, or vertebrae, of the spine are shock-absorbing structures called intervertebral discs. If one of these discs bulges out of its normal position, or bursts, an affected dog will have suffered an intervertebral-disc protrusion, often referred to as a 'slipped disc'. This most commonly occurs either in the neck or around the middle of the back.

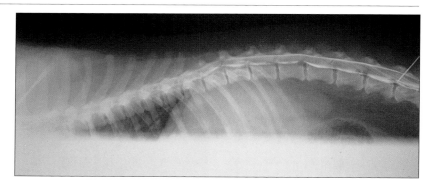

Causes

The shock-absorbing properties of intervertebral discs may be lost due to changes in their internal structure. This may occur in some breeds – such as the dachshund – between eight months and two years of age, or later in life as a result of the same developmental disorder that causes them to have short, bowed legs.

In other breeds – such as the beagle and the spaniel – changes to the structure of the discs may occur later in life for unknown reasons, typically when the dogs are between eight and 10 years old.

Whatever the cause, the result is that failing discs may be squeezed out from between the vertebrae, because of stresses that they would normally withstand. Some discs may even burst, and more than one disc may fail at the same time.

A normal disc may protrude quite unexpectedly in a medium-sized or large dog of any age.

Is it serious?

This is one of the most painful conditions to affect dogs and may cause paralysis, so all cases require emergency care.

Dogs at risk

Disc protrusions in the neck rarely occur in dogs who are less than two years old, and most commonly affect the beagle, corgi, dachshund,

An obvious 'dent' in the middle of the spine indicates a protruded disc; this dog was unable to use his hindlegs.

doberman pinscher, Jack Russell terrier and all types of spaniel.

Disc protrusions in the middle back occur most commonly in young dogs of breeds with bowed legs, and in medium-sized or larger dogs of any age.

Action

If your dog exhibits any of the symptoms described, contact your vet centre immediately.

Your vet will analyse your dog's symptoms carefully and will give him a thorough examination. He or she may also take X-ray pictures of his spine, and may refer him to a specialist vet centre for further tests and treatment.

Treatment

This will depend on the location and number of discs involved, and on the severity of symptoms, but at its simplest may just involve strict rest for three to four weeks and anti-inflammatory medicines.

In some cases, surgery may be required to remove the pressure of the damaged disc or discs on the nerves of the spinal cord.

COMMON SYMPTOMS

An affected disc normally bulges or bursts towards the spinal cord. The symptoms shown will depend on the location of the disc and the degree to which it affects the nerves of the spinal cord. The most common symptoms result from severe pain, and may include the following:
• Tautness of the muscles along the back of the spine.
• Crying and howling when the dog is handled.

• General apprehension
• A hunched posture
• The disc may put pressure on the spinal-cord nerves, causing loss of control of one or more limbs.
• In a disc protrusion affecting the neck, the dog may be reluctant to lower his head to eat or drink.
• A disc protrusion in the middle of the back may cause incontinence, due to the dog's loss of control of his bladder and bowels.

Rupture of the cranial cruciate ligament

The cranial cruciate ligament is one of two tough bands of tissue within a dog's knee. These link the main bones involved in the joint – the femur and the tibia – and help to prevent any unwanted movement.

Rupture of the cranial cruciate ligament is a common condition in dogs, and is often an underlying cause of osteoarthritis of the knee joint in older dogs (see pages 46–7).

Causes

Rupture of the cranial cruciate ligament may be caused by sudden trauma to the knee joint, as might occur when a dog plants a hind foot in a rabbit hole and stumbles.

However, most ruptures are thought to result from structural changes in the ligament itself, which gradually weaken it and make it vulnerable to breaking under the stresses and strains of normal movement.

Is it serious?

This condition does not appear to be especially painful at first, but it must be taken seriously as almost all affected knee joints will develop osteoarthritis (see pages 46–7).

COMMON SYMPTOMS

• An affected leg is carried off the ground and slightly bent; at first, there is usually very little swelling of the knee joint.
• Without treatment, a dog may begin to use the leg after a week or so, but will stand with his toes just touching the ground.
• Muscle wastage may be evident within a week of the rupture.
• A clicking sound may be heard when the dog walks.

Dogs at risk

All dogs are at risk, but those who are 'knock-kneed' or have bowed hindlegs may be more vulnerable.

Action

If left untreated, the lameness may seem to improve over six to eight weeks as the knee joint thickens in response to the instability inside it. However, this alone is usually insufficient to stabilize the knee, and symptoms are likely to recur – especially in large dogs – after vigorous exercise.

If your dog shows the typical initial symptoms of a ruptured cranial cruciate ligament, do not ignore them simply because he does not appear to be in great pain. You must take him to see your vet, as the longer this condition is left the more difficult treatment may be, especially in large dogs.

Your vet will examine your dog carefully, in order to rule out any other hindleg conditions such as hip dysplasia (see pages 50–1).

Rupture of the cranial cruciate ligament causes a characteristic instability in the knee joint, which can be demonstrated by special manipulation: your vet may need to sedate your dog to relax his leg muscles to do this (see page 96).

Treatment

Small, light dogs generally respond well to strict rest for a minimum of six weeks. Painkilling medicines are not normally needed.

Most large dogs will require surgery, involving one of several techniques to stabilize the knee.

A support bandage will then be applied to the affected leg for the first week after surgery, and severe

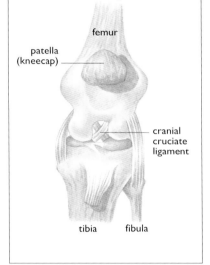

A DOG'S KNEE JOINT

A dog's stifle, or knee, is a complex biomechanical 'hinge'. The joint is stabilized by several tough ligaments, including the so-called cruciate ligaments.

femur

patella (kneecap)

cranial cruciate ligament

tibia   fibula

---

exercise restriction is essential for a further five to six weeks. After that, you should be able gradually to increase your dog's exercise. At first he will be very stiff on the leg, but he should be using it normally within three months of surgery.

Aftercare

If your dog is at all overweight, you must follow the dietary advice of your vet (see also pages 82–3), as a dog who is obese will be more likely to damage his repaired knee again when he starts exercising. He will also run a greater risk of damaging the ligament in his good knee during his convalescence, when that leg will have to carry more than its fair share of weight.

Skin and coat

Skin and coat problems are the most common reason for dogs in the UK being taken to vet centres for medical attention. If your dog suffers from a condition of this kind, it is very important that his symptoms are investigated thoroughly in an attempt to identify the underlying cause. It is sometimes relatively easy to use drugs to control the major symptoms of many skin conditions – such as scratching – but, unless the cause is found and specific treatment given where possible, symptoms will soon recur once treatment is stopped.

Scratching and skin-nibbling

Dogs like to scratch themselves occasionally, just as we do; they also nibble at their coats with their teeth now and again. However, excessive scratching and/or skin-nibbling is abnormal.

Causes

Scratching and skin-nibbling are symptoms of underlying skin conditions, rather than conditions in their own right. As you might imagine, dogs scratch and nibble at themselves in an attempt to relieve any irritation that they feel in their skin. The most common underlying causes include parasite infestations (see pages 58–61), hypersensitivity reactions (see pages 56–7), and pyoderma (see pages 62–3).

Flank- and foot-nibbling appear to be fairly common symptoms of anal-sac disorders (see page 36).

Is it serious?

Never ignore the symptoms of excessive scratching and nibbling shown by your dog, as they will almost certainly be significant. In addition, if the underlying cause stays unidentified and untreated, your dog may rapidly damage his skin and cause further serious and possibly long-term problems.

Dogs at risk

All dogs are at risk of skin conditions that cause irritation.

Action

If your dog begins scratching and nibbling, first check for evidence of fleas in his coat (see page 59), as their feeding and breeding habits will be the most likely cause. If you cannot find any fleas or flea droppings, but you have not treated your house or your dog recently for fleas, you should do so (see page 59).

If your dog continues to scratch and nibble skin, or if his symptoms deteriorate rapidly, arrange for him to be examined by your vet.

Your vet will consider the history of your dog's symptoms carefully, and will examine him thoroughly. To try to identify the underlying cause or causes of the skin irritation, he or she is likely to carry out tests such as analysis of skin-scrapings or intradermal skin testing (see page 57).

Treatment

You should not expect your vet to administer a miracle cure at your dog's first appointment. It is really very important that the underlying cause of the problem is identified, and this may take some time, depending on the tests that need to be carried out.

It may be possible to produce a dramatic improvement in your dog's symptoms by administering certain drugs – notably steroids. However, these drugs represent a symptomatic treatment, and not a cure, so your vet will only resort to them if there is no specific cure for the underlying cause of the problem, if the cause cannot be found, or to help break the 'itch-scratch-itch' cycle while treatment for a curable cause takes effect.

This is because, unless the cause of your dog's condition can be identified and properly resolved, he will almost certainly start to scratch and nibble at his skin once again as soon as treatment with the drugs is stopped.

COMMON SYMPTOMS

The signs of scratching and nibbling are obvious. For reasons that are unclear, the degree of skin itchiness, or pruritus, experienced by a dog may be influenced by his mental state as well as by other sensations acting on the skin such as heat, cold, touch and pain. For instance, itchiness is often worst at night and when a dog is stressed.
• A simple test to find out whether your dog feels itchy is to scratch his side with your fingertips. If his hindleg starts rhythmically beating on the ground and he makes self-satisfied moaning sounds, he may have a problem.
• A dog may also show symptoms associated with any underlying cause, such as reddened skin, hair loss or skin scaling (dandruff).

Alopecia

Alopecia is a complete or partial lack of hair in areas in which it is normally present. Although a completely unnatural condition, alopecia in some breeds, such as the Mexican hairless and the Chinese crested dog, is considered normal by some dog authorities.

Causes

A dog who is suffering from an 'itchy' condition such as a parasite infestation (see pages 58–61) or a hypersensitivity reaction (see pages 56–7) may develop areas of baldness through his excessive nibbling, grooming and scratching attempts to relieve irritation.

Other causes of alopecia include hormonal conditions such as hypothyroidism (an abnormality that can cause complete hair loss over an affected dog's entire trunk, sparing only his head and other extremities), dermatophytosis (an uncommon fungal condition of the skin known as 'ringworm'), and abnormalities of hair growth or moulting. Pinnal alopecia affects a dog's ear flaps, and is especially

common in dachshunds. Seasonal flank alopecia is an abnormality of hair moulting that results in baldness on the flanks of certain dogs of particular breeds, including the Airedale terrier, British bulldog and doberman pinscher.

Is it serious?

Alopecia may be associated with a serious underlying condition such as a hypersensitivity reaction or hypothyroidism, so all cases of baldness should be taken seriously until proven otherwise.

NORMAL HAIR GROWTH AND MOULTING

• Hair grows in cycles. An individual hair grows until it reaches a set length, governed by a dog's genes: this depends on his coat type and the hair's position on his body. After a variable period (affected by factors such as daylight length and ambient temperature), the hair is shed.
• A healthy dog does not go bald when he is shedding his coat, or moulting, because no two hairs that are near each other on his body will be at the same part of the growth cycle at the same time.
• Most dogs moult once in the spring when they grow a thinner, coarser coat, and again in the autumn when they grow a thicker, woollier coat.
• Hair grows at different rates on different parts of the body. In some places on some dogs, it can grow up to 7 mm (⅜ in) per week.

Dogs at risk

The risk depends on the cause of the condition (see left).

Action

If you spot an obvious bald patch on your dog, or if he develops a sparse hair-coat, you should take him to your vet. If he is scratching and grooming himself excessively, do so as soon as possible.

Your vet will examine your dog thoroughly to try to identify the cause of the alopecia. This may involve investigations including blood tests for hormonal disorders, tests relating to specific underlying causes (such as hypersensitivities), and skin biopsies (see page 93) to look for microscopic abnormalities in the anatomy of the skin.

Treatment

Some of the underlying causes of alopecia – such as infestations of parasites, hypersensitivity reactions and hormonal disorders – can be controlled or treated medically. Other problems – such as seasonal flank alopecia – tend to improve without treatment, but will usually recur. There is no known treatment for pinnal alopecia.

COMMON SYMPTOMS

• A dog suffering from an 'itchy' condition may develop alopecia on the parts of his body that he can scratch, chew, lick, nibble or rub. Affected areas may contain broken hairs, and the skin may be inflamed and sometimes infected.
• Alopecia due to other causes does not normally lead to irritation, unless complicated by other skin disorders.
• In seasonal flank alopecia, the skin may be darker than normal.

Alopecia is affecting the thighs and tail of this doberman pinscher.

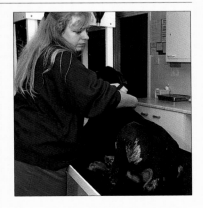

Hypersensitivity reactions

Hypersensitivity reactions involve a complex chain of events that takes place when a dog's immune system over-reacts to the presence either in or on his body of an alien substance. Hypersensitivities are often referred to as allergies.

Dogs may suffer from a number of hypersensitivity conditions that affect the skin, of which the two most common types (in the UK) are flea-bite hypersensitivity and atopy. Other conditions include hypersensitivity to certain foods and allergic-contact dermatitis. A dog may suffer from more than one hypersensitivity at the same time.

FLEA-BITE HYPERSENSITIVITY

In regions that have cold winters, fleas are normally a seasonal pest only during the warmer months of the spring, summer and autumn. However, fleas may be active all year round in warm environments.

Causes

Flea-bite hypersensitivity is caused by a dog's immune reaction to the saliva injected into his skin by fleas during their feeding activities.

Is it serious?

A severe hypersensitivity reaction can be extremely distressing for a dog, and he may cause further serious skin conditions such as pyoderma (see pages 62–3) due to his efforts to relieve irritation.

Dogs at risk

This condition can affect any dog. The symptoms usually first appear in hypersensitive dogs when they are from three to five years old.

Symptoms only rarely occur in puppies under six months of age.

Action

If your dog starts to show any of the symptoms described, take him to your vet as soon as possible.

Your vet will consider the history of your dog's symptoms in detail and will then examine him thoroughly, paying particular attention to any skin lesions that he may have, as well as looking for evidence of fleas or their droppings (see pages 58–9).

However, do not be surprised if your vet cannot find evidence of a flea infestation on your dog: 15 per cent of dogs with proven flea-bite hypersensitivity are flea-free at the time of examination.

The above investigations may suggest a flea-bite hypersensitivity, in which case your vet may decide to begin treatment straight away. However, if there is any doubt, a special skin test will be necessary (see opposite, above).

Treatment

This will involve the following:
• Rigorous flea-control, especially in your dog's environment.
• The use of anti-inflammatory medicines (ideally, for as short a time as possible).
• The use of other medicines, including special shampoos, to treat any infections or other skin disorders that may have occurred as a direct result of the condition.
• Techniques aimed at trying to desensitize your dog may be tried, but these are often unsuccessful.

FOOD HYPERSENSITIVITY

This is an immune-system reaction to specific proteins found in certain food items. Most affected dogs are hypersensitive to one or more items: beef, dairy products, chicken and chicken eggs, wheat, corn and soya have all been implicated. This condition is less common than flea-bite hypersensitivity or atopy.

COMMON SYMPTOMS

A flea bite on a hypersensitive dog causes a raised bump on the skin that lasts for about three days and will be intensely itchy. A hypersensitive dog who is regularly bitten by fleas is likely to lick, chew and scratch at his skin and, as a result, may develop the following further symptoms:
• Hair loss over affected parts of the body, particularly the lower back and base of the tail.
• Areas of stubble where hairs have been broken off by scratching.
• Symptoms associated with a skin infection, such as pyoderma or seborrhoea (see pages 62–3), which may develop if a case of flea-bite hypersensitivity is left untreated.

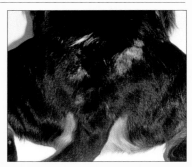

The hair loss on both sides of this dog's lower back, and the moist area of skin on the left, are the result of his attempts to relieve the irritation caused by flea-bite hypersensitivity.

ATOPY

Atopy is a hypersensitivity reaction of the skin to certain substances, or allergens, in the environment. As the allergens are normally inhaled, atopy is sometimes called allergic inhalant dermatitis.

Causes

The allergens that may cause a dog to react include house dust and house-dust mites, human or other animal dandruff, pollens, fungi and moulds.

Dogs at risk

Atopy may be more common in bitches than in male dogs. The following breeds are also especially prone to the condition:
• Beauceron
• Belgian tervuren
• Boxer
• Cairn, West Highland white, Boston, Scottish and wire-haired fox terriers
• Chinese shar pei
• Dalmatian
• English setter
• Golden retriever
• Irish setter
• Labrador retriever
• Lhasa apso
• Miniature schnauzer
• Pug
• Shih tzu

Action

If you notice any of the symptoms described, you should arrange an appointment for your dog to see your vet soon as possible.

To confirm that atopy is the cause of the problem, your vet will consider the history of your dog's symptoms carefully, and will then examine him meticulously. He or she may wish to carry out specific tests, such as a coat-brushing (see pages 58–9) or a skin scraping (see page 61), in order to rule out a parasite infestation.

If your vet believes that your dog is suffering from atopy, he or she is likely to wish to carry out intradermal skin tests to confirm those substances to which your dog may be hypersensitive (see above, right). Blood tests may also be appropriate (see page 93).

Treatment

Natural desensitization in dogs is uncommon, but the symptoms of atopy in nine out of 10 individuals can be controlled. Treatment will include avoidance of substances to which your dog is hypersensitive, by taking the following steps:
• Keeping your dog out of the house, or shut away in a room, during cleaning and vacuuming.

• Not allowing him to sleep on carpets or stuffed furnishings.
• Keeping him indoors when mowing the lawn.
• Avoiding dusty dog foods.
• Limiting the number of plants and cut flowers in his environment.
• Rinsing him off thoroughly after he has had a walk in fields of tall grass or weeds.
• Keeping him indoors at dawn and dusk during periods of high pollen counts.

A dog with atopy should be bathed every one to two weeks, using hypoallergenic shampoos, to prevent dry skin and to remove substances to which he may be hypersensitive. Anti-inflammatory creams or ointments, and anti-inflammatory medicines (including natural-oil preparations), may help to relieve itchiness.

Treatments aimed at making the dog's immune system less reactive to the substances causing the atopy may also be given. Treatment is normally required for life.

Prevention

Susceptibility to atopy is thought to be hereditary, so an affected dog should not be used for breeding.

Flea infestation

In most countries, flea infestations are a very common underlying cause of skin complaints in dogs. There are about 3000 types of flea, of which the type most frequently found on dogs is the cat flea.

Causes

Despite what many people think, fleas spend most of their lives in the environment, not on dogs. An adult flea will jump on to a dog to feed, biting through his skin in order to suck blood.

A number of fleas are likely to have the same idea at the same time. While they are on the dog, they will frantically mate and the females lay hundreds of eggs. In just a few days, the adult fleas die. The eggs drop to the ground, and in under two weeks a flea larva hatches from each egg.

Over the next few weeks to months each larva grows, feeding on mould, crumbs, human and other animal dandruff, and even tapeworm eggs (see pages 32–3). It then spins itself a cocoon shell before building itself an adult body. As an adult, it can survive starvation for about eight months waiting for a dog (or a cat) meal to come along. When the flea senses vibration nearby, it begins to jump. The whole lifecycle may take up to two years.

Is it serious?

A flea infestation can be extremely debilitating for those dogs who are hypersensitive to flea bites (see page 56). Fleas are also a common source of tapeworm infestations to some dogs (see pages 32–3).

COMMON SYMPTOMS

Fleas are visible to the naked eye, but it is unusual to notice them in the environment except in the case of a very bad infestation.

Even if you cannot identify adult fleas on your dog, you may spot the telltale droppings, containing dried blood, that they will leave in his coat (see below).

Other symptoms of an infestation of fleas may include the following:
• Your dog may twitch his skin from mild irritation as the fleas scurry about, or may groom and scratch himself more than normal.

• A hypersensitive dog (see page 56) is likely to feel extremely itchy and to indulge in excessive scratching, licking and fur-nibbling. He may have tiny raised, red lumps on his skin, as well as skin scaling (dandruff).
• Symptoms that are associated with an intestinal-tapeworm infestation (see pages 32–3). Flea larvae may eat tapeworm eggs in the environment, and a dog may swallow a flea that contains an egg while he is grooming himself. As he digests the flea's body, immature tapeworms will be freed to develop in his intestines.

Dogs at risk

All dogs are at risk. Your dog may pick up fleas from other dogs, cats or animals such as hedgehogs and rabbits, or from the environment in which any of these animals live.

Action

Regularly check your dog's coat for fleas and their telltale droppings.

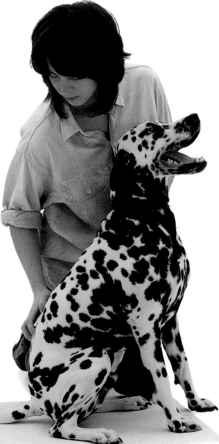

To check for fleas, sit your dog on paper and brush his coat with your fingers (left). Pick up the debris with damp cotton wool: any flea droppings will dissolve to reveal dried blood (below).

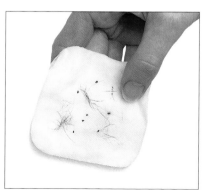

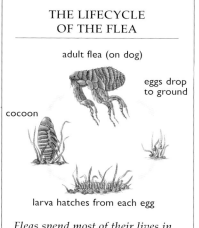

THE LIFECYCLE OF THE FLEA

adult flea (on dog)

eggs drop to ground

cocoon

larva hatches from each egg

Fleas spend most of their lives in the environment, only jumping on to animals to feed and breed.

To do this, sit him on a sheet of white paper and brush the fur on his back with your fingers (see opposite). Specks of dirt and debris will fall on to the paper.

Moisten a cotton-wool pad with water, and dab it over the paper to pick up the specks, then wait a few minutes. Look closely at the cotton wool: any dried flea droppings will have begun to dissolve, and you will see brown stains developing from the dried blood inside them.

If you identify flea droppings, you should treat your dog and your house with appropriate

ZOONOSIS

Most houses containing pets will have a resident population of fleas. If a hungry flea cannot find a dog or a cat, it may jump on to you to feed. Having sucked some blood, it will jump off again and resume its wait for a canine or feline meal. If you are sensitive to their bites, you will be well aware of the fleas in your house.

insecticides, and instigate a flea-prevention campaign (see below).

A dog who has a severe skin reaction will need urgent medical treatment, as he will quickly make his skin condition worse through scratching and excessive grooming.

Symptoms associated with a flea infestation are very similar to those of other skin conditions, so your vet should examine your dog very thoroughly. He or she is likely to carry out the coat-brushing process (see opposite and below, left) and, if your dog shows symptoms of hypersensitivity reactions, may carry out intradermal skin tests (see page 57) before implementing appropriate treatment.

Your vet may also need to treat any self-inflicted skin problems such as pyoderma (see pages 62–3).

Prevention

• Regularly vacuum-clean and then wash all your dog's bedding, and vacuum around your house (an insecticidal collar in the cleaner bag may help to kill any adult fleas that hatch out inside it).
• Regularly spray around your house with an insecticide designed to kill adult fleas. Some products will also stop flea eggs from developing, and only need to be used a few times a year.
• Regularly treat your dog, and any other dogs and cats who live with him, with high-quality insecticidal products made for them (ask at your vet centre about the best products to use, and about the flea situation in your area).

Flea treatments are available in many forms: as collars, powders, shampoos, foams, skin drops, preparations to give by mouth (see pages 101–2) and sprays (below). The ways in which they work differ from product to product, and no one product is perfect for all dogs and in all circumstances. Some products are unsuitable for young puppies or pregnant bitches. Ask at your vet centre for advice on the most appropriate treatments to use on your pets and in your home (the most up-to-date products may only be available from your vet centre).

Infestation of other skin parasites

A dog's skin and coat may become home to several parasitic creatures in addition to fleas. Biting lice and some mites may live on a dog's skin, and survive by eating flakes of skin and debris, together with secretions produced by the skin.

Sucking lice and ticks live on the skin, and use their needle-like mouthparts to pierce through it to feed on blood and other fluids.

Other parasites of dogs, such as demodectic and sarcoptic mange mites, actually spend all or part of their lives within the skin itself.

LICE

The two types of lice to affect dogs, sucking lice and biting lice, are small, flattened, wingless insects. They are spread through direct contact between dogs, or on shared grooming tools and bedding. These lice can be seen by the naked eye, although a magnifying glass makes their identification easier.

Infestation with lice is called pediculosis and is uncommon in the UK and in the USA, perhaps because lice are easily killed by routine insecticidal treatments used to control fleas (see page 59). Dogs living in very overcrowded or unhygienic conditions, those with matted and ungroomed coats, and those who are old or ill are most likely to suffer from pediculosis.

Some dogs carry lice without showing any adverse symptoms, but on other dogs these parasites may produce the following:
• Itchiness
• A 'mousey' smell to the coat.
• Seborrhoea (see page 63)
• Anaemia (in a heavy infestation of sucking lice).
• Other symptoms caused by self-trauma due to irritation .

TICKS

Ticks are eight-legged creatures that are related to spiders. A dog may pick up ticks on his coat by brushing against plants that are infested with them.

The types of ticks that may affect a dog will depend on where he lives. In the UK, for instance, the most common tick parasites of dogs are the so-called 'castor-bean' or 'sheep' tick, and the 'hedgehog' tick. These have hairless or short-haired, leathery bodies and spend their lives in the environment, only visiting dogs or other animals for a few days in the spring or autumn in order to feed.

'Sheep' ticks are visible to the naked eye, but their bodies are often mistaken for small warts or cysts when their heads are buried in a dog's skin. They become most obvious when their bodies swell with sucked blood.

Through their feeding activities, certain ticks may spread serious infections, and may also cause the following symptoms:
• Localized skin irritation
• Anaemia (in a heavy infestation)
• Some ticks in Australia and the USA may cause paralysis.

A tick in a dog's skin is most obvious when it has fed and its leathery body is filled with the blood of its victim.

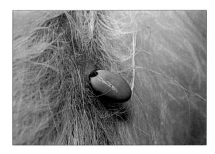

MITES

Mites are tiny creatures that, like ticks, are related to spiders. The following are all mites that affect dogs in the UK.

Cheyletiella mites

These spend their whole lives on the outer surface of a dog's skin. Dogs normally become infested through direct contact with other infested dogs. An affected dog may not feel itchy, but will suffer from severe and obvious dandruff. As a result, infestation with this mite is sometimes referred to as 'walking dandruff'. Cheyletiella mites will also bite people.

Sarcoptic mange mites

These creatures mate on the surface of a dog's skin, and the females tunnel their way into it to lay their eggs. Transmission is generally via contact between dogs. Infestation causes very severe irritation, and the skin often becomes spotty and crusty, especially on the ear flaps, elbows, down the legs and over the chest bone, or brisket. Sarcoptic mange mites will also bite people.

Demodectic mange mites

These may be found in small numbers in the normal skin of a healthy dog. They only cause disease when they are present in large numbers, or on dogs with immune-system disorders. These mites live within the hair follicles, and spend their entire lives on dogs or other animals. They can cause a number of diseases, the most common of which is called juvenile onset demodicosis. This typically occurs in puppies of three to 12 months, and results in bald, inflamed patches of scaly skin.

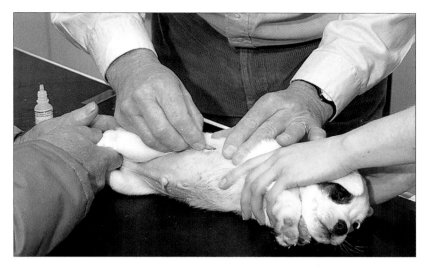

Ear mites
(See page 21.)

Harvest mites
These are common in grassland, especially on very chalky ground. Only the bright orange, young mites are parasitic to dogs, cats and other animals – including people – when they emerge in late summer and autumn. In some dogs, the presence of harvest mites causes very marked irritation of the feet.

FLIES
The adult forms of many flies may lay their eggs on the warm, wet skin of a dog who is debilitated, suffering from a skin wound or has a urine-soaked coat.

The larvae that develop from the eggs may cause severe skin inflammation and tissue damage. Infestation with fly larvae is called myiasis or 'fly strike'.

Is it serious?
The effects of skin parasites on a dog may vary: for instance, they may be fairly minor in some cases of pediculosis caused by a lice infestation (see opposite, below),

In a skin scraping, a scalpel blade is used to obtain a sample of surface skin layers for microscopic examination.

but very severe in an infestation of sarcoptic mange mites.

Action
If you think that your dog may be suffering from an infestation of parasites, if his coat appears in any way unusual or if he shows signs of skin irritation, take him to your vet as soon as possible.

If you cannot identify for certain the presence of parasites on your dog but you think that they may be there, do not carry out treatment at home, using insecticides, until your vet has made a diagnosis.

If you identify fleas, treat them accordingly (see pages 58–9). To remove a tick from your dog's skin, first dab it with a piece of cotton wool wetted with an appropriate insecticide. (Ask at your vet centre for advice; some flea sprays also kill ticks.) Leave the tick for a few minutes to die, then grasp it near the skin with a pair of tweezers, rotate it through a quarter turn and 'unplug' it by pulling gently. Do

not snatch at the tick, or you will be very likely leave its head firmly embedded in your dog's skin: this could result in inflammation and possibly an infection.

In order to confirm the identity of any skin parasite, your vet will examine your dog carefully. He or she may also carry out one or more specific tests – such as obtaining scrapings of his skin, or samples of hair and dandruff – for detailed investigation under a microscope.

Treatment
All dogs with parasite infestations need prompt and very thorough treatment. In most cases this involves the use of appropriate insecticides to kill the parasites. Medicines may also be needed to control symptoms associated with self-inflicted skin damage and infection. Individual ticks and fly larvae must be removed by hand.

Prevention
If you live in an area known to be tick-infested (your vet centre will advise you on this), you will be able to incorporate measures to control ticks into your routine flea-prevention campaign (see page 59).

Grooming your dog regularly will enable you to spot symptoms associated with skin parasites as soon as they appear, so that you can take prompt action.

ZOONOSIS

Many of the skin parasites that affect dogs will cause occasional symptoms in people. If you have any unusual bite marks on your body, contact your doctor. You should also arrange for your dog to be checked for parasites by your vet, even if you do not think he is showing any symptoms.

Pyoderma •

Pyoderma is the term used to describe any bacterial infection of the skin, and is common in dogs.

Causes

In healthy dogs, certain bacteria live at the skin surface and within the hair follicles, and help to resist skin infection by harmful bacteria.

Most cases of pyoderma occur as a result of other disorders, such as conditions affecting the skin's structure, or immune-system problems that allow the normally harmless bacteria to proliferate and cause disease. The following are common types of pyoderma:

Acute moist dermatitis • Also known as 'hot spots' or 'wet eczema', typical symptoms are inflamed, moist, painful, smelly sores that are most common on long-haired dogs in hot and humid weather. In some cases the cause is never identified, but this kind of pyoderma often seems to be linked with self-trauma due to other conditions such as parasite infestations (see pages 58–61), hypersensitivities (see pages 56–7), anal-sac disorders (see page 36) and even otitis externa (see pages 20–1).

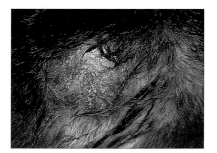

If it is left untreated, this small area of acute moist dermatitis will spread very rapidly over the affected dog's skin.

Skin-fold pyoderma • Skin folds cause an increase in humidity and temperature at the surface of the skin, promoting bacterial growth. Common sites include the lower lip (especially in the spaniel), face folds in dogs with flat muzzles (such as the British bulldog and Pekinese), and folds around the vulvas of overweight bitches. Affected skin folds are inflamed, moist and smelly.

Impetigo • Also known as 'puppy pyoderma', this slightly deeper-seated infection occurs in the non-hairy skin of three- to 12-month-old puppies. Small, pussy spots develop and then rupture, leaving yellow scabs.

Pruritic superficial folliculitis • This extremely itchy condition is particularly common in short-coated dog breeds such as the boxer, dachshund, dalmation and doberman pinscher. Its underlying causes may include seborrhoea (see opposite), hypothyroidism (see page 55) and hypersensitivity reactions (see pages 56–7). An affected dog may develop swellings or bumps on the skin and/or areas of alopecia (see page 55) where the skin is reddened. The skin may appear to peel back in a circle around individual lesions.

Callus pyoderma • This is a deep infection of thickened skin that covers bony prominences – such as the elbows – of large, heavy dogs. Infection may occur due to repeated damage to these areas, or due to other causes such as hypothyroidism (see page 55) or immune-system disorders.

Acne • This condition affects puppies of three to 12 months old. It involves the formation

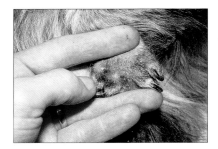

This case of interdigital pyoderma was caused by a penetrating grass awn. The skin between the toes is very inflamed.

of pustules on the face and chin, which often resolve without treatment as the puppy matures.

Interdigital pyoderma • This deep infection affects the skin between the toes. It may occur for various reasons, including the following:

• The presence of foreign bodies (such as grass awns, thorns or wood splinters).

• Matted fur between the toes

• Due to skin damage after walking on rough surfaces or contact with irritant chemicals such as tar and oil.

• Skin hypersensitivities (see pages 56–7) may involve the feet.

• The feet may be the site of fungal infections and parasite infestations – particularly demodectic mange and harvest mites (see pages 60–1).

• Highly-strung dogs and those with anal-sac disorders may bite their feet, causing skin damage. This condition may affect one or more feet, which may be swollen and inflamed. There may be a bloody discharge, especially from cyst-like swellings that are associated with certain foreign bodies (especially grass awns).

Is it serious?

Deep-seated infections can be hard to resolve. They may cause great discomfort, and possibly scarring.

Action

A dog may rapidly turn a minor case of pyoderma into a major one through scratching and licking at his skin, so the sooner your vet is involved, the better. He or she may perform blood tests, skin scrapings (see page 61) or intradermal skin tests (see page 57).

Treatment

Your vet will prescribe antibiotics to clear the infection and reduce inflammation, and may treat any lesions topically with antib shampoos or ointment. Treatment for any underlying cause – such as thyroid supplementation in a case of hypothyroidism – will also be carried out. If a cause is not found, symptomatic treatment may be the only option. Thorough parasite control will help to prevent the recurrence of pyoderma.

Seborrhoea ⚕

A dog's skin is a very dynamic organ: its outer layers are renewed about every three weeks as dead skin cells are lost and replaced by new cells. Seborrhoea is a condition in which the very delicate balance between cell loss and replacement is affected, causing the overall skin thickness to change and the dead cells to become obvious.

Causes

Most cases of seborrhoea occur due to other conditions that affect the structure of the skin, the way it renews itself, or the secretions it produces. These include:
• Hormonal conditions such as hypothyroidism (see page 55) and diabetes mellitus (see pages 76–7).

• Nutritional disorders such as deficiencies, excesses or imbalances relating to glucose, essential fatty acids, proteins and various trace elements and vitamins in the diet.
• Infestations of skin parasites (see pages 58–61).
• Hypersensitivity reactions (see pages 56–7).
• Pyoderma (see opposite).
• Low humidity and high ambient temperatures.
• Over-vigorous grooming, or excessive bathing using harsh or inappropriate shampoos.

Dogs at risk

Seborrhoea is thought to be a hereditary condition in certain breeds, particularly the American cocker and English springer spaniel, basset hound and West Highland white terrier.

Action

If your dog shows the symptoms described, take him to your vet. Do not groom your dog beforehand.

Confirming seborrhoea is fairly easy; more difficult is identifying the cause. To try to do so, your vet will consider your dog's symptoms and examine him thoroughly, and may carry out tests including a skin scraping (see page 61), blood tests, intradermal skin tests (see page 57) and analysis of skin and hair samples (see page 93).

Treatment

The main aim of treatment is to correct any identified underlying cause. It may also involve:
• Bathing using special shampoos (this may be needed indefinitely).
• Antibiotics, if the seborrhoea has led to pyoderma (see opposite).
• Adding animal fat and vegetable oil to your dog's diet.
• Anti-inflammatory medicines in low doses (for very inflamed skin).

Prevention

This involves parasite control (see pages 58–61), regular grooming, a balanced diet and avoidance of hot, dry surroundings.

COMMON SYMPTOMS

Precise symptoms will vary from dog to dog, even if seborrhoea is due to the same cause. It may affect the whole body, or specific areas, and typical symptoms may include the following:
• Skin flakiness and greasiness
• Skin inflammation (dermatitis)
• Areas of alopecia (see page 55)
• An abnormal odour to the coat
• Itchiness

This severe seborrhoea is due to untreated atopy (see page 57).

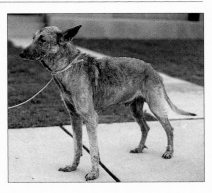

Claw conditions

Claws, or nails, are dead, horny structures on the ends of each of a dog's toes. The special skin that makes them has a very rich blood supply, and the claws of some young dogs up to two years old have been recorded as growing as much as 1.9 mm (1/16 in) per week. In older dogs, the claws may grow at half that rate.

Claws are very useful parts of a dog's anatomy. They can help him to hold objects, will provide grip when he is moving and can even be used as weapons. Of the many nail disorders that may affect dogs, overlong claws and broken claws are the most common.

Causes

A dog's claws grow all the time, and under normal circumstances they are constantly worn down through wear and tear. Overlong claws are caused by insufficient wear and tear, and dogs who are inactive because of age, illness or the laziness of their owners are most likely to suffer from them.

The outer two claws on each paw and the dew claws (see opposite, below), are those that are most likely to be affected.

Damage to the claws is often the result of digging or scrambling, and is more likely to occur if the claws are overlong.

Is it serious?

Overlong claws will affect the way a dog walks, and will make his feet more prone to other injuries such as sprains. If left untreated, the claws may eventually grow around in a circle and bury themselves into the toe pads, causing severe pain.

Dogs at risk

All dogs are at risk, but inactive dogs or those who only exercise on soft ground are more likely to suffer from overlong claws.

You should check the condition and length of your dog's claws once a week during his routine health-checks (see pages 8–9). This golden retriever's claw is very healthy and the perfect length.

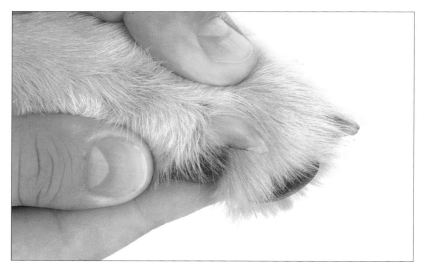

COMMON SYMPTOMS

Overlong and broken nails are obvious on examination. Other signs may include the following:
• Lameness (see pages 44–5) due to toe pain, especially in the case of a broken claw.
• Resentment at any handling of the feet.
• When a dog walks on hard surfaces, overlong claws are often heard before they are seen.

Action

If you think that your dog's claws may be too long, ask your vet, a veterinary nurse or a professional dog-groomer to look at the claws for you. If they are too long, he or she will clip them.

If your dog's lifestyle means that this problem may recur, ask for a demonstration of how to clip your dog's claws properly and safely yourself. Many owners are very reluctant to clip their dogs' claws from the fear that they may make the claws bleed, or that they may hurt their dogs. However, there is no guarantee that a claw will not bleed even if your vet or a dog-groomer clips them, as judging the correct length can be very difficult, especially if the claws are jet-black.

If you do cut a claw and it bleeds, you can stop the bleeding with a styptic pencil. Any pain associated with claw clipping is usually due to the use of blunt or inappropriate clippers, which squeeze rather than cutting cleanly. Few dogs enjoy having their claws clipped, but those used to having their feet examined regularly as part of routine health-checks (see pages 8–9) will normally tolerate

TRIMMING YOUR DOG'S CLAWS

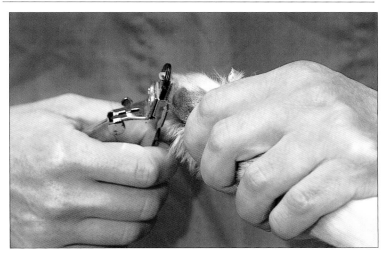

Before attempting to clip your dog's claws, ask your vet or a veterinary nurse, or a professional groomer, to demonstrate the technique (above).

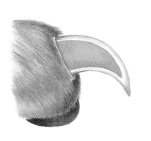

In a white claw, the sensitive pink 'quick' is obvious (right); the claw should be cut just beyond the point where the pink colour fades. Black claws are more difficult to judge.

Treatment

If your dog has a claw that has been seriously damaged, it may be necessary for your vet to remove the broken part – or even the entire claw – surgically. This procedure will be carried out under a general anaesthetic (see pages 96–7).

Prevention

To prevent your dog's claws from growing too long, part of his daily exercise regime should include walking on hard surfaces, such as concrete or tarmac.

You should keep a close eye on the length of all your dog's claws as part of his routine health-checks (see pages 8–9), and trim them – or have them trimmed – as necessary. Remember that it is much easier to remove the little tips of claws on a regular basis rather than large sections every now and again.

During these checks you should pay particular attention to your dog's dew claws (see below), as these do not make contact with the ground during normal movement and are therefore the most likely claws to grow too long.

the experience. However, some dogs resent the procedure so much that they have to be sedated.

With a broken claw, if the tip is hanging off but the claw is not bleeding and does not look raw, you may be able to clip it free. The toe may be painful, however, so you should muzzle your dog first and ask someone to restrain him properly for you (see pages 98–9). If the claw is badly damaged, and particularly if it looks raw or is bleeding, bandage the affected paw (see pages 108–9). This will stop the claw from moving, and will make your dog more comfortable until you can take him to your vet.

DEW CLAWS

Most dogs have five toes on each foreleg (four weight-bearing toes and a dew claw), and four weight-bearing toes on each hindleg. Some dogs also have a dew claw on each hindleg. The front dew claws are the equivalent of our thumbnails and, if you watch the way your dog manipulates objects such as toys, you will see how useful they are.

Unfortunately, some dogs have their dew claws removed as young puppies, to prevent the claws being damaged in later life. In my opinion, this routine removal of dew claws is barbaric and quite unnecessary.

Normal, healthy dew claws are no more likely to be injured than any other claw (most damaged dew claws are overlong when they are damaged: they are not worn down like the other claws, and so need to be trimmed regularly).

If you plan to obtain a puppy, make sure that his dew claws will not be removed, or, if you intend to breed from your dog, do think very carefully before subjecting the litter of puppies to this procedure. It may be traditional for some dog breeds to have only four front toes, but that does not make it right.

Kidneys and bladder

A dog's urinary system consists of the two kidneys and bladder, the ureters (small tubes) that connect them, and the urethra through which urine is emptied from the bladder. Dogs are vulnerable to a number of conditions that affect different parts of the urinary system. Simple urinary tests can be extremely useful in identifying disorders of the kidneys and bladder, so expect your vet centre to encourage you to bring along a urine sample from your dog at his or her annual health-check (see pages 66 and 112).

Cystitis

This condition is inflammation of the internal lining of the bladder.

Causes

Cystitis is generally caused by bacterial infections. The urethra, which carries urine away from the bladder during urination, is inhabited by bacteria. These find their way there from the skin and bowels, due to the normal and inevitable contamination of the area around the open end of the urethra within a bitch's vulva, or at the end of a male dog's penis. Every time the bladder is emptied, these bacteria are washed away.

However, any disorder that reduces the frequency or degree of urination may lead to cystitis. The main reasons are blockage of the urethra: for instance, as a result of urolithiasis (see page 69) or by tumours; nerve disorders affecting bladder control; or a dog being given insufficient opportunity to urinate at normal intervals. Other causes include bladder trauma, cancer (see pages 74–5) and diabetes mellitus (see pages 76–7).

Is it serious?

'One-off' infections will usually respond well to therapy; other causes such as cancer and diabetes mellitus are much more serious.

Very occasionally, a bladder infection may lead on to a serious infection of the kidneys.

Dogs at risk

Bitches are at greater risk than male dogs of bladder infections.

Action

If your dog shows any symptoms described, take him to your vet.

As well as examining your dog, your vet may pass a tube called a urinary catheter up the urethra to check that it is not blocked: this is an easy procedure in males, but bitches often need to be sedated. Your vet may also collect a urine sample via the catheter for testing (see page 93), or may obtain one through your dog's skin and bladder wall with the aid of a syringe and needle.

Your vet may take X-ray pictures of your dog's urinary system, and may also carry out an ultrasound investigation (see page 92).

COMMON SYMPTOMS

- Urination 'accidents' indoors
- More frequent passing of small volumes of urine.
- Blood-tinged urine
- Discomfort on urination (male dogs who normally cock their legs may squat to urinate).
- Abdominal pain when the dog is picked up or handled.

Treatment

If your dog seems to have a simple bladder infection, your vet will prescribe antibiotics. If the cystitis is due to another cause, treatment will be given as appropriate.

Aftercare

Encourage drinking by adding slightly salty gravy to your dog's food, and provide the opportunity for him or her to urinate frequently.

Prevention

Allow your dog to urinate several times a day, in order to encourage the flushing of bacteria out of the bladder and urethra.

A tool for collecting urine samples consists of a scoop with a handle. Your vet centre should supply you with a device similar to this one if necessary.

Chronic renal failure

A dog's kidneys have several vital functions, but they are best known for their role in removing the waste products of protein-processing from the body, and for maintaining the body's water levels and the chemical substances dissolved in that water. The filter-like working parts of the kidneys are called nephrons; each kidney contains about 400,000 of these.

The most common kidney condition, or renal disorder, to affect dogs is chronic renal failure. In most cases this is an irreversible condition in which over 500,000 of a dog's 800,000 nephrons are permanently damaged or destroyed.

Causes

About half of all cases of chronic renal failure in dogs are thought to be due to complex diseases that affect the blood-filtering unit attached to the end of each of the nephrons. Other causes include long-term kidney infections or inflammation and thickening of the internal structure of the kidneys, anatomical defects present at birth, and cancer (see pages 74–5).

Is it serious?

Chronic renal failure is a condition that is progressive and irreversible, so the outlook is poor.

An affected dog may suddenly go into a life-threatening state of acute renal failure, in which the remaining kidney nephrons that are still functioning effectively all shut down at the same time.

Dogs at risk

All dogs are at risk of chronic renal failure, but its symptoms do not normally appear until an affected dog is over five years old.

Action

If your dog is drinking more than usual, or shows any of the other symptoms described, arrange for him to see your vet as soon as you can. If possible, take with you a sample of the first urine that your dog passes that morning: your vet centre should supply a collecting device (see opposite, below).

The initial symptoms of chronic renal failure – particularly that of increased drinking – are common to a number of conditions.

In order to confirm renal failure, your vet will evaluate your dog's symptoms and will examine him thoroughly. He or she will analyse a urine sample, and will perform blood tests. Taking X-ray pictures and carrying out an ultrasound examination may also be necessary (see pages 92–3).

COMMON SYMPTOMS

A dog is able to survive without showing any symptoms of renal failure, even when the whole of one kidney and one-third of the other have been destroyed by disease. The symptoms that are associated with chronic renal failure generally develop fairly slowly, and they may include the following:
• An increased volume of urine, due to the dog's inability to concentrate his fluid waste.
• Increased thirst to compensate for the increased water loss.
• General illness and debility (vomiting, diarrhoea, depression, anorexia, weight loss, bad breath) as a result of inability to remove toxic waste from the body.
• Anaemia
• Bone abnormalities

Treatment

The treatment of chronic renal failure has two aims: to control the progress of any underlying cause, and to help the dog to compensate for the loss of the kidney nephrons that are no longer functioning.

In-patient care • If your dog is very ill, he will need intensive care. This will almost certainly involve fluid administration by intravenous drip (see page 95), and special nursing.

General management • If your dog is eating and drinking well and is not seriously dehydrated, your vet is likely to implement a treatment plan that is based on rest, stress avoidance and a diet containing restricted amounts of protein, phosphorus and sodium. It will be possible to prepare a diet of this type yourself from fresh, high-quality ingredients, but a convenient option may be to use a prepared diet for dogs with chronic renal failure (see page 104). It is usually best to feed on a little-and-often basis. Fresh water must be freely available.

Medication • Your vet may also prescribe medicines to correct abnormalities in your dog's body chemistry, to treat anaemia and to control symptoms such as vomiting (see pages 28–9). Treatment is for life. Your vet will regularly reassess your dog and adapt his treatment as necessary.

Aftercare

At home, you must keep your dog warm, rested and stress-free, and monitor his progress by weighing him and recording his inputs and outputs (see pages 110–11).

Urinary incontinence

Urinary incontinence is defined as the involuntary passage of urine. It is much more common in bitches than it is in male dogs.

A bitch who is suffering from a urinary-tract infection, such as cystitis (see page 66), may appear to be incontinent if she is prone to urination 'accidents' indoors, but she will be conscious of having emptied her bladder, and will have done so voluntarily. A bitch or a male dog who has true urinary incontinence will pass urine without being aware of doing so.

Causes

Voluntary urination involves co-ordination between the muscular wall of the bladder, two muscular urethral valves and abdominal pressure. The most common cause of urinary incontinence in bitches is thought to be incompetence of the urethral valves, which normally prevent urine flowing away from the bladder between urinations. In the majority of cases this is thought to be due to low blood levels of the hormone oestrogen, or to an abnormally positioned bladder with a short urethra.

Less common causes of urinary incontinence include defects in the urinary system (in which the 'plumbing' that carries urine from the kidneys bypasses the bladder), or genital abnormalities that allow urine to pool in an unusual site, such as the vagina. Cancer (see pages 74–5), urolithiasis (see opposite), a nerve disorder such as the protrusion of an intervertebral disc (see page 52) and prostate-gland disorders in male dogs (see page 73) are also causes of urinary incontinence.

The rough collie is one of several breeds that seem to be especially prone to developing urinary incontinence.

Is it serious?

Most cases will respond to medical treatment (at least initially), but anatomical abnormalities may require surgery.

Dogs at risk

Medium-sized and large bitches seem most prone to incontinence due to incompetent urethral valves. The condition appears to be most common in the doberman pinscher, Irish setter, miniature poodle, old English sheepdog, rough collie and springer spaniel.

In one study, nine out of 10 bitches with urinary incontinence were spayed, and half of these had developed the condition within one year of being neutered.

Action

If your dog is showing any signs of incontinence, take him or her to see your vet as soon as possible.

Your vet will examine your dog and will carry out tests – including urine analysis – to confirm true urinary incontinence. Next, to try to identify the cause, he or she may carry out X-rays and ultrasound investigation (see page 92), as well as genital and rectal examinations.

Treatment

A specific cause may need surgery: for instance, to anchor a bitch's abnormally positioned bladder deeper within her abdomen.

If a cause is not found, your vet is likely to 'test-treat' your dog or bitch with medicines aimed at improving the effectiveness of the urethra as a seal to stop urine flow between normal urinations. These medicines may include oestrogens for bitches, testosterone for male dogs or another drug for either sex called phenylpropanolamine.

Some cases do not respond to all logical treatments; these dogs will need nursing to avoid dribbled urine soaking into the coat and causing serious skin inflammation. Cutting the hair and smearing the genital area with petroleum jelly will help (see also pages 106–7).

Prevention

Urinary incontinence in spayed bitches is one reason why many vets recommend neutering after a bitch's first heat (see page 71).

COMMON SYMPTOMS

Depending on the cause, typical symptoms of urinary incontinence may include the following:
• Continuous urine dribbling.
• Intermittent dribbling of urine when the pressure inside an affected dog's abdomen is raised, such as when he or she lies down, is excited, barks, coughs or jumps.

Urolithiasis

This is a condition that causes the development of a mineral 'stone' or 'stones' called urolith(s) within a dog's urinary system. They usually form in the bladder.

Most uroliths consist of struvite (mainly made up of magnesium ammonium phosphate), and may reach a considerable size. Other uroliths contain cystine, oxalate or urate as their main ingredient.

Causes

Urolith formation is thought to be influenced by several factors. These include the quantities of particular salts dissolved in a dog's urine, the presence of substances in the urine that may encourage salt crystals to develop from these dissolved salts, and the ability of formed crystals to remain within the bladder long enough to form uroliths (perhaps by sticking to the bladder wall or because of sluggish urine flow).

The majority of cases involving struvite uroliths are associated with specific urine infections.

Is it serious?

Bladder uroliths may not cause problems until they are extremely large. However, in some cases they

COMMON SYMPTOMS

Other than in the most serious cases in male dogs (see above), symptoms may be similar to those of cystitis (see page 66), as follows:
• Incontinence, or straining to urinate, in a male dog who has a urolith blocking his urethra.
• Blood-stained urine and obvious discomfort towards the end of a urination, in the case of bladder uroliths in male dogs and bitches.

can completely block the flow of a male dog's urine and lead to acute renal failure (see page 67).

Dogs at risk

Urolithiasis can occur at any age, although most cases arise in dogs of between four and six years old. Commonly affected breeds include the cocker spaniel, dachshund, dalmation, miniature poodle, shih tzu and Yorkshire terrier.

Action

If your dog shows symptoms of this condition, take him to see your vet. If you have a male dog and he is straining to pass urine, contact your vet centre immediately.

If the uroliths are very large, your vet may be able to palpate them. He or she is also likely to pass a catheter (fine tube) up your dog's urethra to check that it is not blocked with a urolith, and may take a urine sample for analysis. X-rays of the bladder and urinary system, and an ultrasound investigation of the abdomen, may also be carried out (see page 92). Your vet's aim will be to identify the precise type of uroliths present.

Treatment

This will depend on the type, size and position of the urolith(s), but common procedures include:
• Surgery to remove oxalate and cystine urolith(s).
• A male dog who has a urolith blockage may need an alternative opening to be created in his urethra to re-establish urine flow.
• In a male dog who has uroliths in his urethra, a technique called hydropropulsion may be used to wash them back into the bladder, where they are easier to remove.

The dalmation, along with some other breeds (see left) appears to be particularly susceptible to urolithiasis.

• Struvite or urate uroliths can be dissolved by special medicines or by the use of specific prepared diets (see page 104) that directly affect the chemistry of the urine.
• Antibiotics may be used to treat any associated urine infection. During treatment, your vet may repeat tests such as urine analysis to monitor your dog's progress.

Aftercare

At home, you must administer your dog's prescribed medicines (see pages 101–2) and follow the dietary advice that you are given.

Prevention

The main preventive measure for a dog who has had urolithiasis is to increase his water intake so that he produces more urine to flush out any developing crystals from his bladder. You can add more water to your dog's food, but he may simply drink less. Alternatively, add small amounts of salt to his diet (on your vet's advice) or feed him on a complete diet formulated to help prevent urolithiasis.

Reproductive system (female)

A bitch's reproductive system includes her two ovaries and the Y-shaped uterus. A bitch who is spayed when she is young (primarily as a birth-control measure) cannot suffer from conditions associated with the uterus or ovaries, as these are removed surgically during the spaying. On the other hand, it is common for unspayed (entire) bitches to suffer later in life from a life-threatening condition affecting the uterus, called pyometra. Many entire bitches also experience physical and mental changes during pseudo-pregnancy.

Pseudo- (False) pregnancy

A bitch who does not conceive during a heat enters a state called pseudo-pregnancy (see below). In some bitches this may go quite unnoticed, while others will suffer from both physical and mental changes almost identical to those that they would experience if they really were pregnant.

Pseudo-pregnancy is a perfectly natural process. For example, all the females in a wild-dog pack will come into heat at the same time, but only the top, or so-called alpha, females normally become pregnant. All the others will go into a state of pseudo-pregnancy, and will simply act as wet-nursing nannies!

Causes

Pseudo-pregnancy is a part of the normal reproductive cycle of a bitch (see below). The mental and physical changes that affect some bitches are thought to be due to a hormone called prolactin.

Is it serious?

During pseudo-pregnancy, some bitches become extremely anxious, as well as aggressively territorial. This kind of sudden mood change in their dogs can often be very distressing to owners.

Those bitches who do show symptoms of pseudo-pregnancy may show progressively more marked symptoms after the end of each heat.

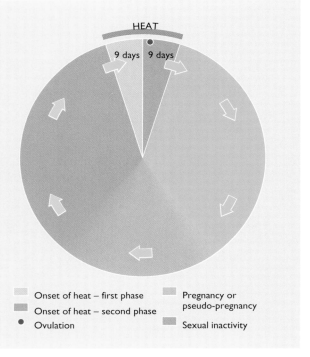

THE REPRODUCTIVE CYCLE OF A BITCH

For most of the year, a mature (unspayed) bitch is incapable of becoming pregnant. However, for a period of about three weeks – generally at intervals of about seven months – all normal bitches come into a heat, or season. During a heat, the reproductive system prepares for mating and possible pregnancy through changes in the levels of certain major sex hormones that may also cause sudden mood changes.

The onset of a heat is marked by the appearance of blood-stained discharge from the bitch's swollen vulva, and lasts for about nine days. At this stage, the bitch will be attractive to males but will not let them mate with her.

As the second phase of the heat begins, the discharge becomes more straw-coloured, and the bitch will soon be at her most fertile. She will usually ovulate (produce eggs) about two days into the second phase, but may allow males to mate with her for another week.

Following a heat, a bitch will either be pregnant or she will enter pseudo-pregnancy. She will then go through a period of reproductive inactivity until her next heat.

This is a simplified view of a bitch's reproductive cycle: start at the beginning of her heat and follow the cycle clockwise. Some bitches have regular heats; others are more erratic.

HEAT

9 days | 9 days

- Onset of heat – first phase
- Onset of heat – second phase
- Ovulation
- Pregnancy or pseudo-pregnancy
- Sexual inactivity

COMMON SYMPTOMS

If a bitch shows any symptoms of pseudo-pregnancy, she will usually do so four to nine weeks after her previous heat. These symptoms may include the following:
• Breast development and the production of milk.
• Nest-building
• Shivering and crying
• Reluctance to exercise
• Mock labour, including straining.
• Emotional attachment towards inanimate objects such as toys.

Action

If your bitch is showing symptoms of pseudo-pregnancy, and you cannot account for her whereabouts throughout her last heat, your vet should examine her to ensure that she is not actually pregnant. If not, and her symptoms are mild, it is probably best to leave her alone.

Your bitch's symptoms should resolve spontaneously in 10 to 14 days, especially if you give her more exercise than normal and deny her the opportunity to be possessive over inanimate objects.

If your bitch has more dramatic symptoms, your vet can treat her by administering hormones by tablet or injection, or sedatives.

Prevention

The only way to prevent symptoms of pseudo-pregnancy is to stop a bitch from coming into heat. In my view, the best option for any bitch who is not intended for breeding is spaying (the surgical removal of the ovaries and uterus). Preventing heats using hormonal drugs is an alternative for bitches who may be used for breeding at a later stage.

Pyometra

This is a complicated infection of a bitch's uterus. It is a progressive condition that is made worse by each heat. In a severe case, the uterus fills with pus and swells to the size that it would be if the bitch were pregnant.

Causes

The bacteria involved may come from the lining of a bitch's urinary system, and may gain entry to her uterus during a heat while the muscular ring, or cervix, that normally seals off the uterus is open. The blood levels of the hormone progesterone rise during ovulation and remain higher than normal in pseudo-pregnancy, and this may somehow encourage the invading bacteria to take hold.

Is it serious?

A severe and advanced case of pyometra is life-threatening.

Dogs at risk

All unspayed bitches are at risk of suffering from this condition, particularly those who have been treated medically for mismating

(see page 119). Pyometra is most commonly seen in middle-aged and older bitches.

Action

If your bitch shows any of the symptoms described, contact your vet centre immediately.

Your vet will consider the nature of your bitch's reproductive cycles and will examine her thoroughly. In most cases, the symptoms of pyometra are so characteristic that specific tests may not be necessary, but if the symptoms are confusing your vet may carry out blood tests, urine tests, X-rays and ultrasound investigations (see pages 92–3). He or she may also take smears of any vulval discharge for analysis.

Treatment

Unless your vet considers that your bitch is too ill to cope with surgery, he or she is likely to recommend spaying her as soon as possible, to remove her uterus and ovaries, as medical treatment rarely effects a cure. Treatment is also likely to include fluids given by intravenous drip (see page 95), and antibiotics.

COMMON SYMPTOMS

Symptoms appear most commonly within 12 weeks of a heat, and are due to an active infection and the release into the bloodstream of bacterial toxins.

In a mild case, an affected bitch may show the following symptoms:
• Relucance to eat
• Reluctance to exercise
• A poor coat
• Other vague signs of general ill-health.
• A mucus discharge from the vulva that persists intermittently after a heat has ended (not in all cases).

Most bitches suffering from pyometra will exhibit more severe symptoms, including the following:
• Anorexia
• Vomiting (see pages 28–9)
• Increased thirst and increased urine production
• Abdominal swelling
• Lethargy
• A discharge from the vulva (not in all cases): this may be cream-coloured or red-brown in colour.
• Excessive licking of the area around the vulva (this may remove any signs of a discharge).

Reproductive system (male)

A male dog may suffer from a number of conditions affecting the main parts of his reproductive system, which consist of the testicles, prostate gland and penis. For instance, the penis or the scrotum (which contains the testicles) may become damaged through accidental injury, while cancer of the testicles is not uncommon in unneutered (entire) individuals. Undescended testicles are fairly common, while the prostate gland is the part of the reproductive system that seems to cause most problems.

Cryptorchidism

A cryptorchid dog has one or both testicles retained somewhere on the normal route along which they descend from the abdomen to the scrotum during early puppyhood. Studies suggest that between one in a hundred and one in 10 male dogs may be affected.

Causes

A dog's two testicles are located in his abdomen at birth, but begin to descend within a week. By the time most puppies are six to eight weeks old, both testicles can be felt in the scrotum. In some cases this may take longer, so a dog cannot be confirmed as cryptorchid until he has reached puberty at five to 12 months (smaller dogs reach sexual maturity sooner than large dogs).

Failure of a testicle to descend as it should may be due to hormonal or physical abnormalities.

Is it serious?

Retained testicles are at greater risk of becoming cancerous. They may also predispose the twisting

---

A RETAINED TESTICLE

This picture represents a male dog lying on his back, with part of the abdominal wall removed to show the normal route by which testicles descend at birth into the scrotum. The testicle on the right has become stuck in the groin. An undescended testicle should be removed as soon as cryptorchidism is confirmed; the other testicle should also be removed (even if it has descended) to prevent the dog from breeding.

kidney

penis

undescended testicle

---

of blood vessels attached to them, with life-threatening consequences.

Dogs at risk

All male dogs are at risk, especially those of the following breeds:
• Border and lakeland terriers
• English cocker spaniel
• Italian greyhound
• Japanese chin
• Miniature schnauzer
• Pomeranian
• Whippet

Cryptorchidism is believed to be an inherited condition, so an affected dog should not be bred from.

Action

If you think that your dog has this condition, take him to your vet.

Your vet may be able to identify a testicle if it is retained in your dog's groin. However, a dog cannot be confirmed as a cryptorchid until he has reached puberty (see left).

Treatment

As cryptorchidism is probably hereditary, your vet will not wish to treat your dog in any way that may disguise his condition by encouraging a retained testicle to descend. Retained testicles are also prone to disease, so your vet should advise removing both of your dog's testicles by castration.

Prevention

A cryptorchid dog should not be used for breeding.

COMMON SYMPTOMS

• A cryptorchid dog will either have one testicle in his scrotum or the scrotum will be empty.
• A retained testicle may still lie within the dog's abdomen, or may have descended to his groin.

Prostate-gland disorders

Every male dog has a single prostate gland that lies at the neck of his bladder and surrounds his urethra (the tube that carries urine away from the bladder). This gland produces a large part of the fluid that a dog ejaculates with his sperm during intercourse.

There are a number of prostate-gland disorders, some of which may occur at the same time. Perhaps the most common of these disorders are the following:

Hyperplasia • This is considered to be a normal and painless enlargement of the prostate gland, and generally occurs when a dog is between six and 10 years old.

Prostatitis • Inflammation of the gland is generally caused by bacteria that have found their way to the prostate gland from the dog's urinary system.

Other causes of disorders include tumours, cysts and abscesses.

THE URINARY SYSTEM OF A MALE DOG

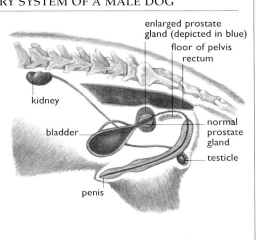

The prostate gland lies within a dog's abdomen, just in front of the edge of his pelvis. The symptoms of prostate-gland disorders, other than acute infections (prostatitis), may not be at all obvious unless the gland is very enlarged. In this case, the gland may put pressure on the wall of the rectum, or may squeeze the urethra within it.

enlarged prostate gland (depicted in blue)

floor of pelvis

rectum

kidney

bladder

normal prostate gland

testicle

penis

COMMON SYMPTOMS

In some cases there may be few (if any) symptoms, but a very enlarged prostate gland pressing against a dog's rectum may cause:
• Constipation (see page 37)
• Ribbon-like faeces
• Straining to pass faeces
   Pressure from the prostate gland on the urethra may produce the following symptoms:
• Straining to pass urine
• Incontinence
Other symptoms may include the following:
• Blood in the urine
• Blood passed from the penis (not associated with urination)
• Pus passed from the penis (not associated with urination)

Is it serious?

In a severe case, a prostate-gland disorder can affect a dog's ability to urinate and to defecate normally. This can lead to serious problems, so all cases need prompt treatment.

Dogs at risk

Prostate-gland hyperplasia only occurs in entire male dogs.

Action

If your dog exhibits any of the symptoms described, you should arrange for him to be examined by your vet as soon as possible.

Your vet should give your dog a thorough physical examination. He or she is also likely to carry out a rectal examination and palpation of the abdomen to feel the outline of the prostate gland, and may pass a polythene tube, or catheter, up the urethra to obtain samples – such as blood or pus – for analysis (see page 93).

Your vet may also decide to take X-ray pictures and to carry out an ultrasound investigation of your dog's abdomen (see page 92).

A biopsy (see page 93) taken from your dog's prostate gland may be required for analysis, especially if he does not respond well to initial treatment.

Treatment

The treatment that is appropriate will depend on the nature of the disorder. In hyperplasia the most effective treatment is castration, but certain hormones or medicines that oppose the effects of normal male sex hormones on the prostate gland may be tried.

Antibiotics – often given as long courses – are used in the treatment of prostatitis, and castration may also help in these cases.

Tumours, cysts and abscesses often require surgical or other sophisticated treatment.

Your vet will wish to re-examine your dog at frequent intervals to check on his progress and response to treatment.

Other important conditions

Various types of cancer, diabetes mellitus (often referred to as 'sugar diabetes'), seizures, umbilical hernias and obesity are all common problems suffered by dogs. Obesity is not only widespread among pet dogs, but – because it causes so much unnecessary suffering – I consider it to be a major animal-welfare problem that should not exist, because it is entirely preventable. Ageing is a natural and inevitable process experienced by those dogs who enjoy a long life, but can bring with it a range of problems and disabilities.

Cancer

Cancer is a very general term used to describe any kind of tumour that is within or on a dog's body.

A tumour is a mass of cells that occurs as a result of normal cells undergoing pointless, persistent division and proliferation. As every cell in a dog's body has the potential to start tumour growth, dogs may suffer from tumours of any tissue or body organ.

Tumours are described as benign or malignant. Benign tumours are typically slow-growing, and do not become intimately associated with the tissues that surround them. They are normally less serious than more aggressive malignant tumours: these are typically fast-growing, irregularly shaped masses of cells which tend to infiltrate the tissues around them and spread to other distant body tissues and organs. Malignant tumours on the surface of the body often ulcerate, bleed and become infected. Almost one-third of all tumours in dogs arise specifically in the skin. The most common of these tumours are the following:
• Benign adenomas
• Mast-cell tumours
• Squamous-cell carcinomas
• Perianal-gland tumours
• Lipomas
   Other common types of tumour include the following:
• Mammary-gland, or breast tumours.
• Soft-tissue tumours
• Lymphomas
• Mouth (oral) tumours
• Bone tumours
• Tumours of the urinary and genital system.
• Tumours of the digestive system

Causes

In the majority of cancer cases, the precise initial cause is never identified. Cells that are apparently normal may spontaneously initiate the development of tumours, or they may be encouraged to do so under the influence of external factors such as viruses, chemicals or radiation. Genetic and hormonal influences may also be involved in some cases of cancer.

It only takes a change in the behaviour of one cell in order to create a tumour.

Is it serious?

All tumours, no matter how small, should be considered serious until proven otherwise by a vet. Benign tumours are not usually fatal, but malignant tumours are invariably fatal if they are left untreated.

Dogs at risk

Cancer is often regarded as a condition that only affects older dogs, but young dogs can suffer from certain tumours. Some breeds may be more prone to developing specific types of cancer than others. For instance, mast-cell tumours are a common type of skin cancer and may affect any kind of dog, but are most common in the boxer.

Action

If you discover a lump or bump on your dog, take him to your vet as soon as possible. Adopting a 'wait-and-see' approach may put your dog's life at risk.

Never ignore any other non-specific symptoms of illness or debility shown by your dog. There is always a chance – especially if your dog is an older individual – that symptoms of this kind may be associated with cancer.

The sooner a tumour has been diagnosed, the sooner your vet can begin appropriate treatment and the better the long-term outlook for your dog will be.

COMMON SYMPTOMS

The symptoms associated with any tumour will depend on many factors, including its location, its size, its interference with normal body processes and whether it is benign or malignant.
• Some tumours, such as those affecting the skin or mouth, may be obvious at an early stage, but the existence of internal body tumours may not be detectable until they are more advanced.

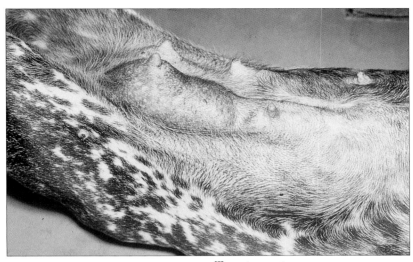

Mammary (breast) tumours are very common in bitches. Approximately half of all such tumours are malignant.

Many cases of cancer are diagnosed by vets during their investigations into symptoms associated with other conditions. For instance, a dog who is lame may turn out to be suffering from arthritis (see pages 48–9), but he could have bone cancer.

Typical ways in which tumours are identified by vets include physical examinations, X-ray and ultrasound investigations, blood tests, and internal examinations of the anatomy using an endoscope (see pages 91–3).

If your vet identifies or confirms a tumour in or on your dog, he or she is likely to carry out further tests to identify its type and size, its involvement with surrounding tissues, and whether it has spread elsewhere. These tests may include X-ray or ultrasound examinations, and taking biopsies (see page 93) or other samples for analysis.

Your vet may undertake these investigations, or may refer your dog to a cancer specialist.

Treatment

Once your vet, or a specialist, has discovered all that he or she can about the tumour, any treatment options can be discussed. Our knowledge of how to treat tumours is growing all the time, and options currently used for cancer in dogs include the following:

Surgery • The aim of surgery is to remove or reduce the size of the tumour mass. Often large areas of tissue have to be removed in association with fairly small tumours, in order to reduce the risk of any tumour cells being left behind. The extent and complexity of surgery will depend on the type, size and location of the tumour, and on its attachment to other tissues.

Chemotherapy • This treatment uses combinations of powerful drugs to kill tumour cells.

Radiotherapy • This is targeted at localized tumours, and is often carried out as part of a treatment regime that involves surgery. To reduce the unwanted side-effects of radiotherapy, a treatment course is normally split up into a number of doses.

Hyperthermia • This involves applying very high temperatures to a tumour to destroy the cells within it. The heat source used is ultrasound or electromagnetic radiation. This kind of therapy is often used in combination with radiotherapy, and is most applicable to skin tumours.

Certain tumours may respond best to individual treatment types, or to combinations of different therapies. Your vet or cancer specialist will select the treatment regime best-suited to your dog's condition.

Aftercare

At home, you must administer any necessary medicines to your dog. He will require special nursing care during his treatment, and your vet or a nurse will advise you of any specific tasks that you should carry out (see also pages 104–7).

No form of cancer therapy offers a guarantee of a permanent cure. If your dog has a serious tumour, the decision as to whether to go ahead with treatment, to let nature take its course, or to end his suffering painlessly through euthanasia (see pages 124–5), may be very difficult to make. It is absolutely essential that you fully understand your dog's problem, and the kind of future that he may be expected to have, with and without treatment.

Listen carefully to your vet's advice, and discuss all the options available so that you can make the best decision for your dog.

WARNING

Although non-cancerous skin cysts are common in dogs, you should never assume that a lump or bump on your dog is a cyst – it may be a tumour. Take your dog to your vet, and let him or her decide.

Diabetes mellitus

Diabetes mellitus is a hormonal condition in which a dog is unable to control the glucose, or sugar, levels in his blood. It is a relatively common condition, and may affect up to one in 100 dogs. There are two types of this condition found in dogs: primary diabetes mellitus and secondary diabetes mellitus.

Causes

A dog's blood-glucose levels are controlled by a hormone called insulin. This hormone is produced by the pancreas, an organ that lies close to the stomach and is also responsible for producing some digestive enzymes.

A dog with diabetes mellitus either suffers from a shortfall in the amount of insulin that his body needs, or he produces enough insulin but his body tissues do not respond to its actions. The result is a higher-than-normal blood level of glucose in an affected individual.

Primary diabetes mellitus is thought to be caused by failure of the pancreas to produce sufficient insulin, as a result of an in-built abnormality of the pancreas or through a deterioration in the pancreas associated with ageing.

Secondary diabetes mellitus is thought to be caused by any of the following factors:
• Destruction of the cells that are responsible for producing insulin, caused by inflammatory diseases of the pancreas.
• The presence within a dog's body of abnormal amounts of other hormones that prevent his tissues from responding to normal levels of insulin.
• The long-term administration of some drugs, such as certain hormones and anti-inflammatory steroid medicines, that prevent the body tissues from responding correctly to the presence of normal amounts of insulin.
• Obesity (see pages 82–3), leading to the overproduction of insulin by the pancreas, and insensitivity of the tissues to its actions.
• An immune-system disorder that causes body tissues to resist the action of insulin.

Is it serious?

If left untreated, a dog suffering from diabetes mellitus will become depressed, vomit, breathe more rapidly than normal, stop passing any urine at all and will eventually end up in a coma and die.

Dogs at risk

Diabetes mellitus most commonly occurs in dogs over eight years old, although cases have been found in dogs of less than 12 months old. Unspayed bitches are three times more at risk than male dogs, due to a rise in blood levels of the hormone progesterone in pseudo-pregnancy (see pages 70–1). Obese dogs are also at greater risk.

The following breeds seem more prone to diabetes mellitus (it may be a hereditary condition in some of the larger breeds):
• Cocker and King Charles spaniels
• Dachshund
• Doberman pinscher
• German shepherd
• Golden and labrador retrievers
• Miniature poodle
• Pomeranian
• Rottweiler
• Samoyed

Action

If your dog shows any of the symptoms described, take him to your vet as soon as possible.

Many of the symptoms of diabetes mellitus are also common to other conditions, so your vet will consider your dog's symptoms carefully and will examine him thoroughly. He or she is likely to carry out blood and urine tests (to look for glucose in the urine), as well as X-ray and ultrasound investigations if necessary (see pages 92–3).

Treatment

The precise treatment regime will depend on the type of diabetes mellitus, and on its cause. Your vet is likely to wish to admit your dog as an in-patient to stabilize his condition. If your dog is very ill, he will need intensive nursing.

Before any treatment begins to control your dog's condition on a longer-term basis, it is essential that you are fully aware of all the responsibilities that you will have to take on (see opposite, above). It is also very important that your vet knows in advance exactly what you are prepared to do.

COMMON SYMPTOMS

The exact symptoms may vary from case to case, but typical symptoms are as follows:
• An affected dog will pass a greater quantity of urine than normal, and may be forced to urinate indoors during the night.
• Increased thirst
• Increased appetite
• Weight loss
• Poor coat condition
• Lethargy
• Cataracts (see pages 12–14)

The following are all common elements of therapy:

Withdrawal of other drugs • Any drug treatment that could be a cause of the condition should be stopped as soon as possible.

Treatment of a specific cause • This will be implemented if a cause (such as another hormonal condition) is identified.

Weight reduction • This is very important for a dog who is overweight (see pages 82–3).

Spaying of a bitch • This should be carried out as soon as a bitch can cope with surgery.

Medication • In some mild cases, medicines may be given by mouth to control the dog's blood-glucose levels.

Insulin • This may be injected on a regular schedule (your vet will show you what to do).

Dietary modifications • A diabetic dog's diet should be high in complex carbohydrates (such as starch and dietary fibre) and low in fat. It should have moderate levels of good-quality protein, but no simple sugars (such as glucose or sucrose). The easiest way to feed a diabetic dog is to offer him a prepared diet proven to help in the management of diabetes mellitus (see page 104). Your vet should give you precise dietary advice for your dog. It is essential that his diet does not vary in consistency or quantity from day to day: every person who comes into contact with your dog must understand that he is not allowed titbits, and that he has set times for his meals.

Exercise • A diabetic dog must be given a consistent daily level of exercise; bouts of strenuous exercise should be avoided.

With careful management, about seven out of 10 dogs suffering from diabetes mellitus can be stabilized

CARING FOR A DIABETIC DOG

You will play an essential role in your dog's care if he has diabetes mellitus. The following is a typical daily routine for an owner of a diabetic dog:

7:00 am
Collect and test urine for glucose.

7:30 am
Give morning feed (⅓ to ½ daily ration). Calculate the amount of insulin to inject, based on urine test and amount of food eaten.

7:35 am
Inject required dose of insulin under the skin.

10:00 am
Controlled walk off the lead for 20 minutes.

2:30 pm
Give afternoon feed (½ to ⅔ of daily ration).

5:00 pm
10-minute walk on the lead.

as in-patients. The majority of these dogs will go on to enjoy a good quality of life for between one and five years, with the help of the committed input and care of their owners and veterinary staff.

Prevention

Many causes of diabetes mellitus cannot be prevented, but the one important step that you can take is to ensure that your dog is not overweight (see pages 82–3).

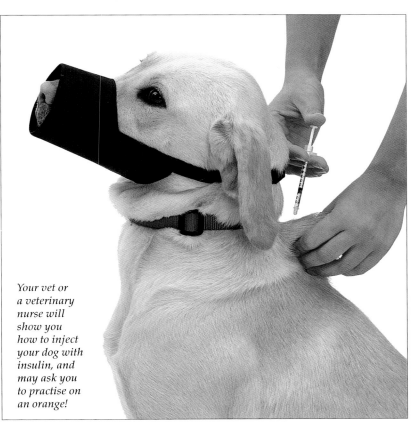

Your vet or a veterinary nurse will show you how to inject your dog with insulin, and may ask you to practise on an orange!

Chronic liver disease

The liver is one of a dog's major organs. It has many vital functions, some of which are: the production of most blood proteins (including those involved in blood-clotting), the conversion of waste products of protein-processing into a substance that can be removed from the body by the kidneys, the processing and storage of carbohydrates and fats, the purification of the blood and the production of bile to aid the process of digestion.

Unusually, the liver may suffer from a sudden, acute disorder such as canine leptospirosis or infectious canine hepatitis (see pages 84–5). Longstanding, or chronic, liver disease is perhaps more common.

Causes

Chronic liver disease in a dog may be caused by anatomical abnormalities present at birth. Other causes are cancer, most commonly due to its spread from tumours elsewhere in the body (see pages 74–5), long-term inflammation, immune-system disorders, or disorders of the bile duct, which empties bile from the liver into the small intestine.

Dogs at risk

Chronic liver disease is most common in older dogs, although anatomical abnormalities may cause symptoms in puppies who are just a few months old.

The Bedlington terrier is prone to a specific kind of liver disorder called copper toxicosis.

Is it serious?

By the time symptoms of chronic liver disease appear, 80 per cent of the liver tissue may have stopped working properly. Sadly, in most

---

COMMON SYMPTOMS

Symptoms are often rather vague, but they may include the following:
• Reluctance to eat
• Weight loss
• Depression
• Lethargy
• Vomiting (see pages 28–9)

• Abdominal swelling
• Excessive thirst
• Jaundice (most obvious as yellowing of the 'whites' of the eyes) .
• Pale faeces
• Diarrhoea (see pages 30–1)
• Abnormal behaviour, such as apathy.

---

cases, the outlook for an affected dog is very poor.

Action

If your dog starts to show any of the symptoms described, or is in any way 'off-colour', take him to be examined by your vet.

Cases of suspected chronic liver disease are often very frustrating to investigate. This is partly because the symptoms are vague, but also because the liver may be affected by or involved in other conditions. There is also no simple test that can be carried out to confirm beyond doubt the existence of chronic liver disease, or to identify its causes.

Your vet will examine your dog and may then carry out blood and urine tests, analysis of any build-up of fluid in your dog's abdomen, X-ray pictures and ultrasound investigations, and a biopsy (see pages 91–3). Exploratory surgery to take a direct look at the liver may also be appropriate.

Treatment

There is no cure for chronic liver disease, so the aim of treatment is to slow down its progression and to control associated symptoms. This may involve the following:
Dietary management • This is the cornerstone of treatment for liver disease. Its purpose is to

reduce the build-up of the waste products of protein-processing, which cause many symptoms of this condition. A diet regime should include the following:
• Easily digested carbohydrates, such as rice (to provide energy)
• High-quality, easily digested sources of protein, such as eggs
• Four to six small daily meals
• Sufficient food to prevent weight loss (some dogs may need force-feeding).
 Commercially prepared diets proven to help in cases of liver disease make a very good and convenient choice (see page 104). Your vet or a veterinary nurse should give you specific feeding advice for your dog.
Rest • Allowing your dog to lead a stress-free life is all-important.
Medicines • These may be given to reduce fluid build-up in the abdomen. Antibiotics and other medicines may be used to treat specific causes or symptoms.

Aftercare

You must keep in close contact with your vet centre: your dog is seriously ill, and must return to his vet for regular check-ups. Sadly, many cases of liver disease are untreatable, and the only option is to end a dog's pain through euthanasia (see pages 124–5).

Seizures

Seizures are often called 'fits' or 'convulsions', and are symptoms of sudden alterations in a dog's brain function. Epilepsy is a condition in which an affected dog suffers from repeated seizures.

Causes

The precise cause of some seizures is unknown, or may be genetic, but others are known to occur for a number of reasons. These include anatomical defects of the brain, infections such as distemper and rabies (see pages 84–5), brain cancer (see pages 74–5) or trauma, severe liver and kidney disorders, and blood-chemistry abnormalities. Puppies suffering from seizures are most likely to have developmental problems, or to be suffering from infections; cancer-related seizures are more common in older dogs.

Is it serious?

As seizures are associated with abnormal brain function, they are extremely serious. If left untreated, epileptic seizures tend to recur at progressively shorter intervals, and some dogs may go into a state of

---

SIMILAR DISORDERS

Other disorders exist that may be confused with seizures, but will be treated differently.
• Fainting is a loss of consciousness in which the muscles are totally relaxed. It is caused by a sudden lack of blood supply to the brain, or by very low blood-sugar levels.
• Narcolepsy is a state of extreme sleepiness. It is sometimes associated with cataplexy, a condition in which a dog collapses and refuses to move. There is no loss of consciousness.
• Idiopathic vestibular syndrome is an acute balance disorder that results in a head tilt. The dog will often walk in a drunken, stumbling fashion and may fall, but will not lose consciousness.
    If your dog shows signs of these disorders, contact your vet centre.

---

continuous seizure activity called *Status epilepticus*, which requires emergency treatment.

Dogs at risk

Epilepsy is most common in the cocker spaniel, collie, golden and labrador retrievers, Irish setter, miniature schnauzer, poodle, St Bernard and wire-haired fox terrier. Most epileptic dogs have their first seizure at between one and three years of age.

Male dogs are more affected than bitches. Unspayed bitches are most likely to suffer from a seizure during a heat (see pages 70–1).

Action

If your dog has a seizure, contact your vet centre immediately. If he is thrashing about, leave him alone. If he is conscious, discourage him from getting up (see also page 119).

Your vet will try to identify the cause of the seizure, by considering your dog's history as well as the seizure. He or she may also carry out (or arrange elsewhere) one or more of the following:
• A physical and neurological examination, involving assessment of the eyes and nerve reflexes.
• Blood/urine tests (see page 93)
• Spinal-fluid analysis
• A brain scan

Treatment

A one-off seizure does not always mean epilepsy, so treatment is not normally initiated unless another attack occurs. If no cause is found, anti-convulsant medicines are usually prescribed (these may be required for life). A dog in *Status epilepticus* needs intensive care.

Aftercare

Your vet will monitor your dog's progress closely. With good care, most epileptic dogs can lead an almost normal life.

COMMON SYMPTOMS

So-called generalized seizures are the most common type, and typically occur in the following three phases:
• The aura: the dog is anxious, fearful or agitated; this phase may last from a few minutes to two days.
• The ictus: the dog falls unconscious with a fixed stare and rigid legs; this is followed by leg-paddling and jaw-chomping. After one to two minutes, he will start to breathe strenuously.
• The post-ictal phase: the breathing quietens, the convulsive movements

slow and the muscles relax. The dog regains consciousness but appears confused. This may last from a few hours to two days, during which the dog may cry, bark, pace around and show abnormal hunger.
    Partial seizures affect only one part of the body, and symptoms may include the following:
• Side-to-side head movements
• Spasm in one or two legs only
• Inappropriate behaviour such as screaming, running or aggression.

Umbilical hernia

A hernia is the protrusion of a piece of tissue through a natural opening in the muscle wall of the abdomen. The most common type is an umbilical hernia, which occurs where a puppy's umbilical cord was attached before birth.

Causes

An umbilical hernia forms due to failure of the body wall to close around the stalk of the umbilical cord. It is almost always due to a flaw in the early development of a puppy's abdomen, but may also be associated with low-grade infection

---

COMMON SYMPTOMS

• An umbilical hernia may become obvious when a puppy is a few weeks old, and will appear as a swelling at his 'tummy button'. Its contents may pop in and out as the abdominal pressure changes.
• Umbilical hernias are normally small and soft, and contain fatty tissue. Larger hernias may contain pieces of bowel or other abdominal structures.

---

of the stump that remains when the umbilical cord is broken.

This condition is more common in certain breeds of dog, so it is possible that genetics plays a part.

Is it serious?

A small hernia is unlikely to cause problems. A larger hernia could be much more serious, as a section of bowel could become trapped inside it and have its blood supply cut off: this is a life-threatening situation that requires emergency surgery.

Dogs at risk

Umbilical hernias are particularly common in the Airedale terrier, Pekinese, pointer and Weimaraner.

Action

If your puppy develops a small swelling at his tummy button, ask your vet for his or her opinion when you take the puppy for a development check. If he suddenly develops a large swelling, contact your vet centre immediately.

An umbilical hernia is normally very straightforward to diagnose on physical examination. If your

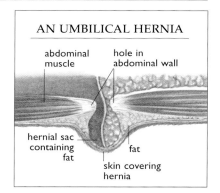

AN UMBILICAL HERNIA

abdominal muscle — hole in abdominal wall — hernial sac containing fat — fat — skin covering hernia

dog has a large umbilical hernia, your vet may carry out some tests such as X-ray investigations, in order to establish its contents.

Treatment

Small hernias often resolve of their own accord as puppies grow up. Those that remain are usually small and do not need treatment, or, in bitches, can be repaired during spaying. A large hernia should be surgically repaired as soon as possible to prevent complications.

If your puppy's hernia is left untreated, you should keep an eye on it for any increase in size.

Growing old (ageing)

Dogs have been known to live to the great age of 29, but the average canine lifespan is perhaps nearer to 12 years. Small breeds tend to live longer than larger breeds; cross-bred and mongrel dogs generally outlive their pure-bred cousins.

A dog's body is a remarkable creation. It can repair itself and has built-in spare parts, but, inevitably, the years take their toll and – as in humans – numerous body changes take place associated with ageing.

You can improve your dog's chances of a long life by providing him with good nutrition, exercise and healthcare, together with special care during the last third of his life: his golden years.

The ageing changes

The following are just some of the common problems that are faced by an older dog:
• Decreased sensitivity to thirst, leading to possible dehydration.

• Less efficient body-temperature control, causing reduced tolerance of heat and cold.
• Increased susceptibility to infections of varying kinds.
• A shallow sleep pattern, leading to irritability.
• Decreased sensitivity of hearing, sight, taste and smell.
• Gum disease and tooth loss
• Decreased saliva production, and difficulty in swallowing.
• Mouth ulcers

- Digestive upsets due to decreases in the efficiency of the stomach and intestines at digesting food.
- Skin abnormalities such as coat dullness, alopecia (see page 55), brittle claws, and a greying muzzle.
- Thickened areas of skin, or calluses, over pressure points such as behind the elbows.
- Decreased kidney and liver function.
- Enlargement of the prostate gland in male dogs (see page 73).
- Cancer (see pages 74–5)
- Muscle weakness
- Arthritis (see pages 46–7) and joint stiffness.
- Weaker and more brittle bones
- Heart failure (see pages 38–40) and high blood pressure.
- Anaemia
- Less efficient delivery of oxygen to the blood (from breathing), causing tiredness on exercise and behaviour associated with senility.
- Decreased numbers of brain cells, leading to slow reaction times and partial memory loss (the first sign of senility often appears as the loss of house-trained toileting habits).

Action

A good diet, sufficient exercise, a stimulating lifestyle and good healthcare from puppyhood will ensure that your dog approaches old age in the best possible shape. From his seventh birthday onwards (or his fifth birthday if he is a giant breed) you should pay particular attention to the following:

Diet • The current view is that an older dog benefits from various nutritional changes, and should be given the following:
- Less calories, because he is less active. If your dog's weight creeps up, cut back his food.
- A more palatable diet, because of his decreased senses of smell and taste (in general, warmed, moist foods are very palatable).
- Reduced amounts of protein, phosphorus and sodium to help him to cope with kidney and cardiovascular (heart and blood-vessel) changes.
- Increased amounts of vitamins A, B1, B6, B12 and E.
- Increased unsaturated fatty acids and zinc, to help maintain healthy skin.
- Small, frequent meals.

Your vet or a veterinary nurse will help you put together a feeding plan for your older dog. Prepared diets for older dogs (see page 104) make a convenient option.

Medical care • By carrying out health-checks on your dog once a week (see pages 8–9) you will be more likely to pick up the

Dogs sleep more as they grow older, but still benefit from regular exercise to keep their bodies fit and their minds alert.

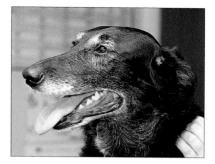

Most dogs are described as geriatric at the age of seven (or five in the case of giant breeds). In terms of general ageing the body of this nine-year-old mongrel is likely to be in a similar condition to that of a 52-year-old person.

early symptoms of common diseases of older dogs such as heart failure (see pages 38–40), arthritis (see pages 46–7), skin conditions (see pages 54–65) and cancer (see pages 74–5). Your vet should also examine him at least twice a year as, if problems in an older dog are identified early, much can be done. It is possible for dogs in their late teens to undergo surgery successfully, and there are even medicines to treat general ageing symptoms such as lethargy and depression associated with senility.

Preventive healthcare • Continue with parasite prevention (see pages 32–4 and 58–61), and keep your dog's vaccinations up to date (see pages 85).

Grooming • Regular grooming is important for coat health.

Dental care • Periodontal disease is a major problem in older dogs, so routine tooth-brushing is vital (see pages 24–5).

Exercise • Even older dogs with arthritis need regular exercise to maintain muscle bulk; it also provides mental stimulation and encourages bowel function.

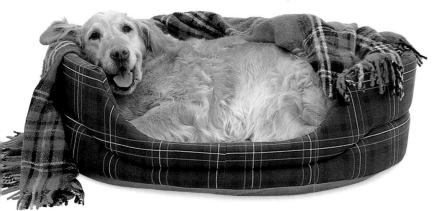

Obesity

Obesity is a condition associated with the accumulation of fat within a dog's body, greater than that necessary for his body to function at its best. It is very common: in the UK, perhaps as many as one-third of dogs seen at vet centres are obese. Obesity may be linked with other conditions, including arthritis (see pages 46–7), diabetes mellitus (see pages 76–7), liver disease (see page 78), breathing difficulties, and heart and circulatory problems.

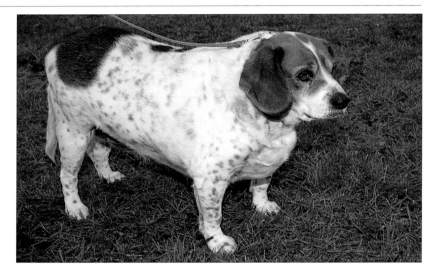

This bitch is obese. Her condition is almost certainly reducing her lifespan, as well as her quality of life.

Causes

The causes of obesity are many and complex, but the underlying problem is simple. If, over a period of time, a dog's diet provides him with more energy (measured as calories) than he burns up, his body will accumulate fat. If this imbalance remains uncorrected, he will become obese.

Owners do not deliberately encourage their dogs to become obese, but many inadvertently do so. The following are some of the mistakes that are commonly made:
• Failing to adjust a dog's meal sizes and total food intake to his actual requirements.
• Ignoring the additional calories supplied by titbits and treats.

• Believing that a large appetite is a sign of good health.
• Offering 'comfort' food when leaving a dog alone.
• Under-exercising a dog.
• Offering many foods in the belief that this will avoid any nutritional 'deficiencies' in a single product.

Other causes of obesity include a dog's genetic make-up, castration or spaying, and other conditions – notably a hormonal disorder called hyperthyroidism (see page 55) – that reduce the rate at which a dog burns up energy.

Is it serious?

Many seriously obese dogs have a miserable quality of life (most owners of formerly obese dogs comment that their dogs have gained a completely new lease of life as a result of losing weight).

There is also little doubt that uncorrected obesity will reduce a dog's life expectancy.

Dogs at risk

All dogs, but especially older and neutered individuals, are at risk. Obesity also appears to be more commonly suffered by certain breeds, including the basset hound, cairn terrier, Cavalier King Charles spaniel, labrador retriever and Shetland sheepdog.

Action

If you know that your dog is overweight, or you think that he may be, take him to see your vet:

COMMON SYMPTOMS

The precise symptoms shown by a dog will depend on the degree of the obesity and on any other conditions involved, but typical symptoms may include the following:
• A covering of fat over the ribs. If your dog is at his ideal weight, you should easily be able to feel his ribs through his skin (if you can see the ribs, he is probably too thin).

• Lack of a definite waistline behind the rib cage when viewed from above.
• A flabby abdominal wall
• A large, pendulous abdomen
• Fatty lumps at the base of the tail and over the hips.
• A waddling walk
• Sluggishness
• Difficulty in climbing stairs, jumping or other physical exertion.

not next week, or next month, but today. Do not avoid taking him from any embarrassment at the fact that you may be partly to blame. Remember that obesity is not just an aesthetic problem, but a serious disease. If your dog is overweight he will be suffering unnecessarily, and you are the only person who can help him.

Your vet will weigh your dog, and will examine him thoroughly to assess the degree of obesity and to establish whether he is suffering from any associated conditions.

He or she may then decide to carry out additional procedures, including blood and urine tests, and perhaps ultrasound and X-ray investigations (see pages 92–3).

Treatment

As a first step, your vet will initiate treatment for any other conditions from which your dog may be suffering, and will then concentrate on the following:

Dietary management • Your vet (or a veterinary nurse) should devise a tailor-made plan aimed at reducing your dog's weight in a controlled manner, taking into account his current diet and lifestyle. Your input is essential, as you will be the one to carry it out: unless you and all your family are committed to your dog's slimming campaign, it is unlikely to be effective. Many vet centres now run slimming clinics where you can talk to other dog-owners in the same situation. Simply adjusting your dog's diet to cut his calories may lead to nutritional imbalances, and his current regime may also have contributed to his obesity, so your vet or nurse is likely to base his new feeding regime on a prepared diet proven to help with obesity (see page 104).

The feeding guide on a dog-food label gives general recommendations only. Your dog will be like no other when it comes to his food, and you will need to adjust the amount that you offer him to match his personal calorie requirements. If you change him to a new food, begin by mixing some of the new food with the old to prevent a digestive upset. After a day or two, offer a daily quantity based on your interpretation of the feeding guide on the product label.

Weigh your dog once a week (see below), and adjust the quantity of his food as necessary.

Exercise management • You may be advised to make changes to your dog's exercise regime straight away, or to wait until he has shed some of his excess weight. Increased activity can help with weight reduction in dogs, but is less significant than calorie control. Your vet or nurse

Your vet or nurse will wish to examine and weigh your dog at least every two weeks, in order to check on his progress.

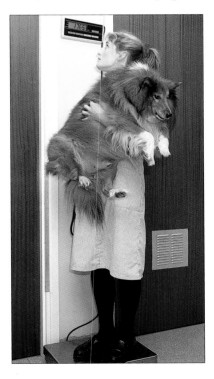

will monitor your dog's progress very carefully. When he reaches what is judged to be his ideal weight, the vet or nurse will offer you further dietary and exercise advice to ensure that he stays that way in the long term.

Prevention

The most important factor here is to plan a sensible feeding regime for your dog from the start. Rather than attempting to make difficult nutritional decisions, ask for advice from someone trained in nutrition, such as your vet or a veterinary nurse. Always think very carefully about what you feed your dog, and try not to make any of the common 'owner errors' (see opposite).

No matter what you feed, you should weigh your dog once a week on the same day and at the same time. This is particularly important when you change his diet or exercise regime in any way, or after he is neutered. If you notice that his weight is dropping, increase his food; if he puts on weight, cut back the food to bring his weight down to his ideal level. It really is that straightforward.

If your dog is a puppy, weigh him frequently. A veterinary nurse should be happy to create a growth chart for him, to compare with one for a normal puppy of his type. By doing so, any feeding mistakes that you make will soon become clear.

Major infectious diseases

All dogs are vulnerable to a number of important diseases, generally called the major infectious diseases. These are caused by organisms – such as certain viruses and bacteria – that may be rapidly passed from an infected dog to healthy dogs. Examples include viral diseases such as distemper, and bacterial diseases such as canine leptospirosis. (For information on contagious respiratory disease, refer to pages 42–3.) The specific infectious diseases to which your dog may be exposed will depend on where you live, and also on his lifestyle: if he regularly visits places frequented by other dogs, his chances of infection will be higher.

Distemper

Distemper is a viral disease that is most common in areas heavily populated with dogs. A dog may inhale the virus during direct contact with an infected dog. The virus may cause damage to the respiratory and digestive systems, and to the skin, eyes and brain.

In a mild case, a dog may be lethargic and reluctant to eat. In a more severe case, he may also have the following symptoms:
• Eye and watery nasal discharge
• Intermittent coughing
• Vomiting (see pages 28–9)
• Diarrhoea, often containing flecks of blood (see pages 30–1).
• Cracked foot pads
• Nervous disorders, such as seizures (see page 79), may occur months or years after infection.

Distemper generally affects dogs under 12 months old. There is no specific treatment available.

Canine parvovirus

A healthy dog may be infected with this virus through exposure to an infected dog, or through contact with an environment or object contaminated by his faeces. In the UK, the virus can survive outside a dog's body for three to six months. In young puppies, it may cause an inflammatory condition of the heart, but this is rare. Enteritis (inflammation of the intestinal lining) is the most common result of infection.

Symptoms may vary, from few – if any signs – of infection to acute diarrhoea and death within 24 hours. However, the most common symptoms include the following:
• Sudden onset of vomiting
• Depression and anorexia
• Very liquid, bloody diarrhoea

Without intensive symptomatic treatment, including antibiotics, a dog may die in 48 to 72 hours (there is no specific cure). A dog who recovers may remain immune to re-infection for life.

Canine leptospirosis

Leptospirosis is caused by different strains of the bacterium *Leptospira interrogans*. One strain mainly attacks the kidneys, while the other two strains attack the liver.

Transmission of the bacteria is normally through contact between individuals, or through a healthy dog's exposure to objects such as food or bedding contaminated by an infected dog's urine.

The most severe infections may cause shock and sudden death. In less severe infections, symptoms may include the following:
• Anorexia
• Vomiting
• Diarrhoea (possibly with blood)
• Dehydration
• Excessive thirst
• Reluctance to move
• Jaundice
• Decreased urine production
• Abdominal discomfort

Aggressive treatment against canine leptospirosis, including appropriate antibiotics, may be successful if started sufficiently early. A dog may pass bacteria in his urine for several weeks after recovering from the disease.

ZOONOSIS

The bacteria that are responsible for causing leptospirosis in dogs can also infect people, and may cause serious disease.

Infectious canine hepatitis

CAV-1 (see right) is passed out of an infected dog's body in his saliva, urine and faeces, and these are all possible sources of infection to another, healthy dog.

This disease is most common in dogs under 12 months old. The virus attacks body tissues, notably the liver, causing inflammation that results in enlargement of the liver.

Most infections are mild, and symptoms may simply include slight malaise and reluctance to eat.

In severe cases, symptoms are clear and may include the following:
• Extreme depression
• Anorexia
• Increased thirst
• Intermittent vomiting
• Abdominal swelling/discomfort
• Sudden death
• Up to one in five dogs develop a temporary cloudiness of the cornea at the front of the eye within two to three weeks of recovery.

There is no specific treatment.

CANINE ADENOVIRUSES

There are two closely related, but quite distinct, adenoviruses that can affect a dog, known as canine adenovirus type 1 and 2.

CAV-1 is a tough virus that can survive outside a dog's body for over 10 days and causes canine infectious hepatitis; CAV-2 is involved in contagious respiratory disease (see pages 42–3).

Rabies

Certain countries, including the UK, are currently free of rabies, but in other regions it is widespread.

Rabies affects a dog's central nervous system. It is most often transmitted by bite, as the virus is present in the saliva of infected animals. The period between the infection and onset of symptoms is usually 10 weeks to four months.

The first symptom is often a change in personality. In one in four infected dogs, symptoms then change to include the following:

• Excitability and restlessness
• Irritability and snapping
• A depraved appetite
• Wandering for long distances

A dog may die in a convulsion or coma, but most develop muscle paralysis and die in seven days.

Prevention

If a dog becomes infected by an organism, his immune system will react to try to destroy it. However, the viruses and bacteria that cause major diseases can be very quick to damage vital body organs, and the immune system may not respond quickly enough to prevent the dog becoming seriously ill or dying.

Vaccination

Vaccination saves life. It improves the speed and effectiveness of a dog's immune-system response to infection, by stimulating it through exposure to harmless amounts of the organism concerned before the dog encounters it for real.

In the UK, a typical vaccination regime may be as follows:

At six to 10 weeks • Distemper, parvovirus, leptospirosis and infectious canine hepatitis (parainfluenza virus may also be included). The vaccines are mixed in a single injection.
At 12 weeks • A repeat of the above. (A puppy should be kept from public places for seven to 10 days after this.)
Four weeks before kennels • Vaccination against *Bordetella* (see pages 42–3).
At 15 months • Parvovirus and leptospirosis (and canine parainfluenza virus). This is repeated every year, with vaccines for distemper and infectious canine hepatitis every other year.

The specific vaccinations that your dog needs will depend on where you live and on the products used.

Vet centres and procedures

A good vet centre will offer you much more than just emergency medical care for your dog. This section offers practical advice on choosing and using your vet centre, and includes background information on some of the most common veterinary procedures that your dog may experience there.

Your dog's health service

If your dog is injured or becomes ill, you will want the best medical attention for him. It is comforting to know that veterinary services are available 24 hours a day, 365 days a year from most vet centres. Even those that do not provide out-of-hours services themselves should make sure that the needs of their patients are properly catered for in an emergency.

The staff at your vet centre will not only treat your dog when he is unwell, but should also provide you with a range of healthcare services including vaccination, parasite control and dental care, as well as very useful information on diet and other aspects of dog care. For the sake of your dog, make good use of them.

Remember that most vet centres are private businesses, and that you will have to pay for most of the services that you use. Veterinary fees are generally extremely good value for money, when you consider the cost of the medical equipment used to treat dogs – much of which is virtually identical to that used on humans – the cost of drugs and the advanced training of veterinary staff.

VETERINARY PROFESSIONALS
A number of key people are involved in the daily work of a typical vet centre, and all will be part of your dog's veterinary team.

Receptionist
The receptionist is normally responsible for booking appointments, handling enquiries, collecting fees and looking after the clients. A dedicated receptionist should be adequately trained to offer general advice about very basic animal healthcare, but should not be expected to provide answers to more serious medical queries.

Veterinary surgeons (Vets)
Having completed their training, many vets choose to concentrate on the care of just one or two types of animal, such as dogs and cats, or horses and farm

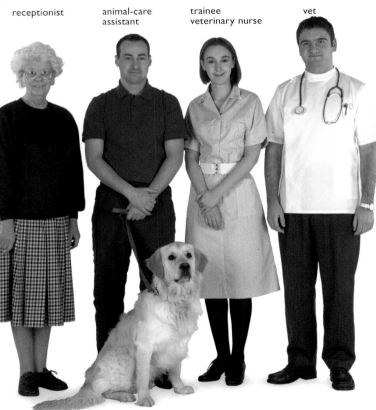

receptionist   animal-care assistant   trainee veterinary nurse   vet animals. However, all vets are qualified to treat any kind of animal – great and small. Your dog's vet will not only be his personal physician but much more besides, including his surgeon, dentist, anaesthetist, pharmacist and perhaps even his psychiatrist!

Many of the routine tasks formerly undertaken by vets are now the responsibility of the veterinary nurses at some vet centres, so that the vets can concentrate on more specialist work. Some vets will go on to gain further qualifications in specific areas of veterinary work, such as dermatology or orthopaedics.

Veterinary nurses

These skilled, highly trained individuals are in my experience the backbone of many vet centres. Just some of the responsibilities of veterinary nurses are to run the operating theatre, to assist the vets with diagnostic, surgical and medical procedures, to look after in-patients, to run the dispensary and to carry out laboratory tests. They may also perform some medical treatments and minor surgical procedures, under the guidance of a vet. Most larger vet centres will employ a number of veterinary nurses.

CHARITY CLINICS

In some areas, veterinary services are offered free of charge, by animal charities, to owners who are on some forms of state welfare. For instance, in the UK the People's Dispensary for Sick Animals has over 40 clinics throughout the country. These clinics are run on public donations, and, in my view, those who use them should be prepared to help with fund-raising if at all possible.

Animal-care assistants

Unqualified, but nevertheless very caring, animal-care assistants help to reduce the workload of the veterinary nurses. Feeding animal in-patients, exercising them and cleaning up after them are all typical duties.

Centre manager

A well-run vet centre can invest in new staff, facilities and equipment that should ensure the provision of an ever-better service for their clients. Some vet centres employ a centre manager, whose responsibilities will include the overall smooth running of the centre and the processing of accounts.

Other staff

Many centres also rely on the help of other staff, including cleaners and handymen. You may not see them, but if your dog ever has to stay in at your vet centre, he will no doubt get to know them briefly, if only for a cuddle!

TYPES OF VET CENTRE

Some vet centres have the facilities and staff to treat animals of any sort – large or small – including horses, farm stock, dogs, cats and other pets; others may concentrate solely on the care of pets.

Vet centres may also be called clinics, surgeries or practices, and the largest and often best-equipped centres are sometimes called veterinary hospitals. By contrast, the smallest vet centres may have only basic equipment and facilities, and may be open for just a few hours each day. Between these two extremes are vet centres of all sizes.

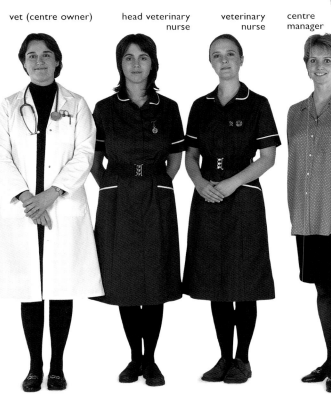

vet (centre owner)   head veterinary nurse   veterinary nurse   centre manager

Get to know your dog's veterinary team. As well as making sure that you and your dog are well looked after, the staff of a good vet centre will be a mine of useful information on every aspect of dog care.

CHOOSING A VET CENTRE

Most people tend to use the vet centre that is nearest to their homes. Your most convenient centre may turn out to be the one best-suited to your needs, but do not simply assume that this will be the case. Investigate the alternatives by following the steps below.

If possible, you should make your initial decision well before you even obtain your dog, so that you can benefit from all the advice available from the centre as you prepare to become a dog-owner.

What to do first

• Look in your local business telephone directory for vet centres, and make a list of all those within 20 to 30 minutes' drive – this is the furthest that you should need to travel in an emergency. Then create a shortlist of those with facilities dedicated to treating dogs.
• Make a quick, unannounced visit to all the centres on your shortlist. On each visit, take note of the ease

A typical vet centre

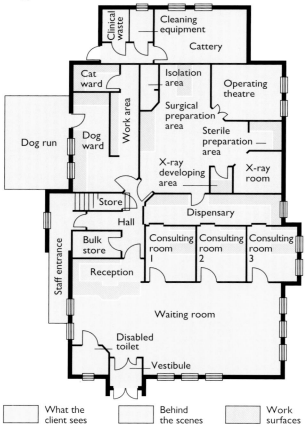

Legend:
- What the client sees
- Behind the scenes
- Work surfaces

of the journey and of access to the premises, the cleanliness of the waiting room and reception area, and the appearance and attitude of reception staff.
• Ask for information about the centre, including details of all the services offered to dog-owners, the centre's opening times and the fees charged (many good centres will produce a brochure). Find out whether it is possible to arrange a tour of the centre. If possible, wait about looking at the notice-board long enough to see how other clients are handled.

What to do next

• Speak to dog-owning friends to obtain their opinions of the centres on your initial list.
• Armed with the information that you have obtained about each centre, and with the views of your friends in mind, prepare a new shortlist. Do not even consider a centre that refuses to give you a guided tour.
• Arrange to view these shortlisted centres. While you are there, try to meet some of the veterinary staff, and take note of their appearance and friendliness.
• Finally, go home, think about everything that you have seen and heard, and then make your decision.

CHANGING YOUR VET

If you move house, you may need to change your vet. In this case, you should select a new vet centre in the same way as is outlined above.

You may also wish to change vet centres if you are unhappy with the service you are receiving. However, before making a hasty decision, do talk through any grievance with a member of staff. It may be that the problem has occurred because of an unintentional breakdown in communications, and it would be a pity to leave a good centre over a misunderstanding.

A SECOND OPINION

If your dog is unwell and his condition does not seem to be improving in spite of treatment, your vet may suggest that he is seen by another vet. You may also arrange a second opinion yourself, although some specialists only take cases referred on by other vets.

THE OWNER'S ROLE

Vets rely on owners to give an accurate account of their dogs' problems, but some owners are perhaps less than truthful about the precise nature, extent and

To give you an idea of what to expect to see when you visit a vet centre, shown here is the interior plan of a typical centre with the facilities for both dog and cat patients.

ACCUSTOMING YOUR DOG TO HIS VET CENTRE

It is not surprising that many dogs actively dislike visiting their vet centres: after all, they may only go there when they are ill or injured, and are then prodded and poked in all the places that hurt most. No matter how kind or considerate your vet or veterinary nurses, your dog may not thank them for some of the things they do to him.

However, by taking your dog to your vet centre for his regular health-checks, the good experiences should outnumber the less good ones. Take him with you every time you visit the centre, even if it is only to pay a bill or to pick up some food, so that going there becomes an accepted and familiar experience for your dog.

longevity of their dog's symptoms from a misplaced fear of being branded as uncaring. Some even try to make key symptoms less obvious by washing and grooming their dogs prior to going to the vet centre!

The aim of all good vets is to help their patients to recover from illness as quickly as possible, and to improve the dog-health knowledge of their owners. They are not interested in judging owners' dog-care abilities. If you are honest and open with them, they will be better able to help both you and your dog.

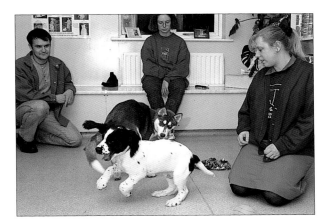

Many good vet centres now run 'puppy parties'. Held over several weeks, these are an excellent opportunity for young puppies to become used to visiting their vet centres, and for owners to learn about the most up-to-date views on dog care.

Health insurance

It is possible to calculate the annual cost of preventive-healthcare procedures such as vaccination and parasite control, but you cannot predict when your dog will be ill or when he may suffer an injury. And, if he does require any veterinary treatment, there is no way of knowing in advance how sophisticated that treatment will need to be, or for how long your dog will need it.

Fortunately, it is possible to insure against the cost of veterinary treatment, and many companies offer a range of policies to suit the needs of dog-owners. For an annual premium, most policies will guarantee to pay all your veterinary fees up to a maximum amount in each year (you will probably have to pay an agreed sum towards each claim).

I would wholeheartedly recommend that you take out health insurance for your dog. I find nothing worse than seeing an owner, distraught about his or her dog's illness or injury, having to cope with the additional worry of how to pay for his care.

When choosing a health-insurance policy, make sure that you read the small print. If you are in doubt about any part of a policy, consult an insurance advisor.

A typical policy may cover the following:
• The cost of veterinary fees for every illness and accident, including physiotherapy, acupuncture and homoeopathic medicines, hospitalization and referral.
• Death following illness: the cost of your dog will be reimbursed.
• Death following an accident: the cost of your dog will be reimbursed.
• Boarding-kennel fees for your dog if you are taken into hospital for more than four days.
• Holiday-cancellation costs if your dog requires emergency surgery up to seven days before or during your holiday, or goes missing while you are away.
• Advertising and reward costs if your dog is lost.
• Loss by theft or straying: the cost of your dog will be reimbursed.
• The repair costs of accidental damage caused by your dog to another person's property.
• Third-party liability in case your dog causes damage or injury and you are legally liable.
• A 'burglar reward' if your dog catches an intruder in your home.

Veterinary procedures

The best way to ensure that you and your dog get the most from the veterinary profession is to familiarize yourself with the services available from most good vet centres. With an understanding of some of the procedures commonly carried out by vets and veterinary nurses, you will be able to make more informed healthcare choices for your dog.

ACCIDENT-AND-EMERGENCY SERVICES

Very few vet centres are open 24 hours a day for their clients to turn up unannounced, but all centres (in the UK) are required by law to provide accident-and-emergency services at all times. If they cannot do so themselves, they will arrange access for their clients to the services of another centre in the area.

Accident-and-emergency procedure

If you need veterinary assistance out of hours, you will normally have to telephone your vet centre. The telephone may be answered by a member of staff on duty, or by an answering machine. The machine will either give you another number to ring, or will ask you to leave a message. It should automatically contact a vet or nurse on duty, and you will then be called back.

One way or another, you will end up speaking to a vet or to a veterinary nurse in person. Remember that, out of hours, the vet or nurse may be unfamiliar to you. Equally, he or she may not know your dog personally, and may not have his records immediately available. Answer his or her questions as accurately as you can, and listen carefully to any instructions that you are given. It is a good idea to write them down.

Depending on your dog's symptoms, your vet may wish to see him. A home visit may be essential in some cases, but if possible the vet will ask you to take your dog to the vet centre. With better facilities there than are available in the back of a car, he or she will be better able to examine and treat your dog.

Try to be sensible about how you use the emergency services of your vet centre, and do not abuse them by telephoning the centre out of hours for minor matters. (For further information on coping with accidents and emergencies, refer to pages 114–23.)

CONSULTATIONS

During working hours, your vet centre should offer the option of an individual consultation with your vet, for him or her to examine your dog or to discuss any other health-related matter. Some centres will also offer consultations with a veterinary nurse for minor procedures or for healthcare advice. 'Open' surgeries are run on a first-come, first-seen basis, but most centres also offer appointments.

What is involved?

The length of a consultation may vary from centre to centre, but it should take at least 15 minutes. In my view, it is not possible to examine a dog, question his owner, make a diagnosis and decide on a treatment in less time than this. Some centres organize surgeries several times a day, and some are open six or even seven days a week.

You should expect to pay a fixed fee for the appointment with your vet, plus extra for any tests, drugs or other products that he or she uses.

A nurse should be on hand to help your vet if necessary. Do not talk to your vet when he or she is using a stethoscope, as you will make it difficult to hear the sounds of your dog's body.

DIAGNOSTICS

Diagnostic procedures are carried out in an attempt to identify the underlying cause of the symptoms that are shown by an ill dog. Many of these procedures – such as examinations using a stethoscope, an otoscope or an ophthalmoscope (see below, right) – may be carried out in your presence by your vet or a veterinary nurse in the consulting room.

Carrying out tests

You should expect your dog to be admitted as an in-patient for procedures such as X-ray investigations, which may require the use of sophisticated equipment or can only be carried out with your dog sedated or anaesthetized (see pages 96–7). If your vet centre does not have the facilities to undertake certain diagnostic procedures, your dog may need to go to another centre to be examined. In this case, your vet should make all the necessary arrangements for you.

The procedures that are most frequently carried out on ill dogs include the following:

Physical examination • A basic physical examination involves a systematic evaluation of a dog's external and internal anatomy through observation and palpation. This procedure may include rectal and/or vaginal examinations.

Temperature-taking • A dog's body temperature is recorded using a thermometer inserted into his rectum. Traditional mercury thermometers and electronic thermometers are both used. The rectal temperature of a normal dog is about 39°C (102°F).

Electronic or traditional mercury-in-glass thermometers are used to measure a dog's core body temperature. Although most dogs tolerate having their temperature taken without fuss, you will be asked to restrain your dog's head during the procedure.

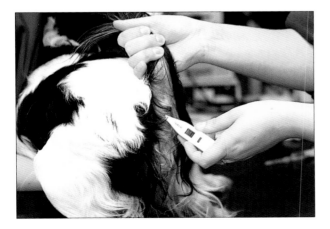

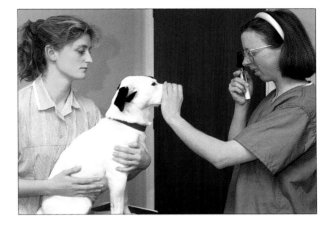

Your vet will use an ophthalmoscope to examine your dog's eyes: this is simply a powerful light source containing a number of different magnifying lenses.

Stethoscope examination • A stethoscope is a device that helps to amplify sounds within a dog's body, such as his heartbeat, the movements of air when he breathes, and the sounds created by the mixing and digestion of food in his stomach and intestines. Avoid talking to your vet when he or she is using the stethoscope, as you will make it difficult for him or her to hear some of the quieter sounds generated from within your dog's body. The heart-rate of a normal dog at rest is 70–140 beats per minute; the breathing rate is 10–30 breaths per minute.

Otoscope examination • An otoscope is an instrument that is used to examine a dog's ears. It has cone-shaped attachments that are designed to fit snugly into ear holes of different sizes, and a built-in light and a magnifying lens provide a clear view of the dark depths of the ear canals. The ear drum of a normal dog appears as a white sheet of tissue across the ear canal.

Ophthalmoscope examination • An ophthalmoscope is an instrument used to examine a dog's eyes. It has a built-in light, a number of filters and a range of lenses to allow a detailed examination of both the internal and external anatomy of the eye. The retina of a normal dog makes a very colourful image when viewed through an ophthalmoscope.

Endoscope examination • An endoscope is a special optical instrument that allows a vet to take a direct and detailed look at parts of a dog's anatomy that are normally hidden from view, such as deep into his airways or down his oesophagus and into his

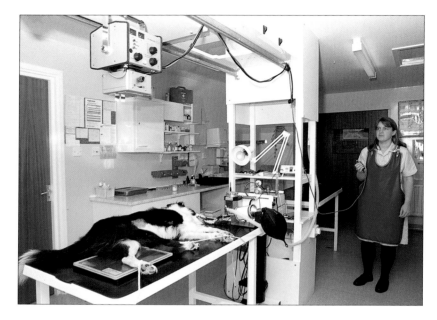

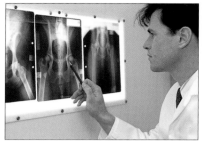

If your dog has an X-ray investigation, your vet will examine the films in detail (above). Ask to see these, and for a full explanation of what they show.

Almost all dogs – with the exception of those who are seriously ill – are sedated or anaesthetized (see pages 96–7) for X-ray investigations. This is because, in order to obtain a clear picture, it is essential that they remain still (left).

stomach. Some endoscopes are rigid tubes; others are flexible pipes whose tips can be moved remotely. A dog will usually be anaesthetized (see pages 96–7) during an endoscope examination.

X-ray investigation • The X-ray equipment found in most vet centres is a smaller version of that used in human hospitals. The pictures that are created by an X-ray machine offer a view of a dog's internal anatomy. Bones are particularly easy to identify, as they show up as white. Other structures are more difficult to visualize, and interpreting X-ray pictures takes both skill and experience. A dog will normally be heavily sedated or anaesthetized (see pages 96–7) during an X-ray investigation.

Ultrasound investigation • If you have had a baby, you will be very familiar with ultrasound machines. Not all vet centres have their own machines, but more and more centres are now obtaining them. Ultrasound machines are highly sophisticated tools that are used to produce complex images of a dog's internal anatomy. Their most obvious and perhaps simplest use is to confirm pregnancy. It is possible to detect pregnancy in a bitch just 16 days after ovulation (the production of eggs) has taken place, but an ultrasound examination is normally carried out at or after day 28 of pregnancy.

Electrocardiography (ECG) examination • An ECG machine records the electrical activity in a dog's beating heart, and is most often used to detect and

identify any abnormalities involving the anatomy of the heart or in the way in which it is working. The procedure involves attaching a number of wires to a dog's skin, and is most often carried out with the dog lying on his side. In some cases, a dog with heart problems may also be fitted with a portable ECG unit; this will record the electrical activity in his heart over a prolonged period.

A basic ultrasound investigation – for example, to detect pregnancy – is carried out with a dog fully conscious and simply restrained by a nurse. It may be possible for you to be present while an ultrasound is carried out on your dog.

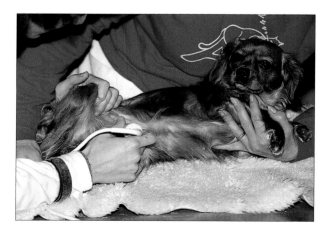

Laboratory procedures

It is likely that – at some point in his life – your dog will have samples taken from him for analysis. Some of the most common procedures are as follows:

Blood tests • These may be carried out for many reasons, such as to assess a dog's body chemistry or the state of his immune system, or to ascertain how well certain vital organs – including his liver and kidneys – are working. Samples of blood are taken either from the cephalic vein in a foreleg, or from the larger, jugular vein in the neck. The blood is then immediately stored in special containers and analysed in a laboratory. Many vet centres have their own laboratories, but send samples to outside laboratories for special tests; other centres may send away all their samples. A number of tests may be carried out on a blood sample at the same time; the results of this are called a blood profile.

Urine tests • These may be carried out for a number of reasons, including to check for abnormalities associated with urinary conditions such as cystitis (see page 66) or urolithiasis (see page 69), or to assess how well a dog's kidneys are working. Glucose is normally absent from urine, but will appear in the urine of a dog who is suffering from diabetes mellitus (see pages 76–7). Your vet may

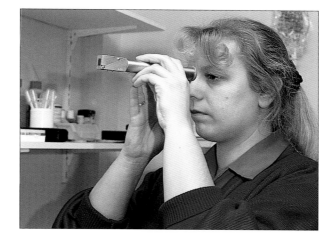

This nurse is measuring the specific gravity (concentration) of a urine sample taken from a dog, using an instrument called a refractometer. The result will give her important information about how well the dog's kidneys are functioning.

In most vet centres the responsibility for running the in-house laboratory, as well as processing blood and urine samples, belongs to the veterinary nurses.

ask you to obtain a urine sample from your dog and, if so, should provide you with a special urine-collecting tool to do so (see page 66).

Biopsy • This is a small sample of a dog's tissue that is removed and sent to a pathologist for examination and analysis of its microscopic structure. A biopsy will be taken under some form of anaesthesia (see pages 96–7), and is a common procedure in the investigation of unidentified growths.

Analysis of fluids • Your vet may send samples of any abnormal fluids taken from your dog – such as pus – to a laboratory so that they can be cultured and examined under a microscope. Any organisms associated with the fluids can then be identifed.

TREATMENT PROCEDURES

Your dog may experience two types of conventional therapy should he become ill: surgical treatments and medical treatments. In many cases, a combined regime involving surgery and medicines is required.

Surgical treatments

Dental descaling, neutering, removing a broken claw, repairing a skin wound, mending a broken bone and removing a growth are just some of the many surgical procedures carried out at vet centres.

Every vet centre should have full surgical facilities on-site, or should have access to them. These will include all necessary general-anaesthetic equipment, an operating theatre stocked with surgical instruments and a post-anaesthetic recovery area. Some centres also have specialist tools such as lasers and freezing equipment. Indeed, the facilities in some of the largest vet centres are very similar to those of human hospitals: much of the surgical and anaesthetic equipment used was developed for use on humans, and then adapted for use on animals.

Surgical instruments and drapes are sterilized prior to use, and are only handled by vets and nurses who have scrubbed their hands with anti-bacterial soaps.

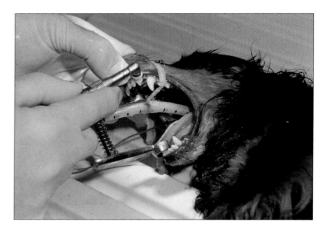

Dental procedures carried out on dogs (see pages 24–5) now account for a large proportion of the surgical treatments that are undertaken at most vet centres.

It is now possible to implant artifical hip joints in dogs, and to carry out open-heart surgery, but the complexity of surgery undertaken at a vet centre will depend on its equipment and on the expertise of its staff. Veterinary nurses may carry out minor surgical procedures such as stitching wounds, and may assist a vet with more major surgery such as spaying a bitch (see page 71). General anaesthetics are usually the responsibility of both a vet and a nurse (see pages 96–7).

Medical treatments

Medical treatments are given to dogs using a variety of methods.

Drugs • These may be given in several ways, including by mouth or topically to the affected part of the body (see pages 101–3), but most of the medicines administered to dogs by vets and veterinary nurses are given by injection, as follows:
• Under the skin, most commonly over the neck.
• Into a muscle.
• Into the bloodstream (most commonly via the cephalic vein in a foreleg).

Fluid therapy • This is the administration of special fluids into the bloodstream via an intravenous drip, and is a common and often life-saving procedure. A dog who is undergoing fluid therapy is often referred to as being 'on a drip' (see also page 105).

Blood transfusion • This may be carried out between dogs when necessary.

DISPENSARY SERVICES

If your dog needs drug therapy, your vet will normally start treatment during a consultation, and will ask you to continue the administration of the drugs at home.

Rather than supplying prescriptions, almost all vet centres run their own dispensary to supply drugs to their clients. The dispensary is usually managed by a veterinary nurse, who will give you advice about how to use any drugs that are supplied.

PSYCHIATRY SERVICES

Advice on coping with the simplest and most common behavioural problems of dogs should be available from good vet centres. Some centres employ individuals – often vets, nurses or zoologists – who have a special interest and expertise in helping owners to resolve more complex behavioural problems. Centres that do not offer such a service should be happy to refer clients to qualified dog-behaviour experts elsewhere.

SERVICES FOR HEALTHY DOGS

Your vet centre is not just there for when things go wrong, but should offer a range of other products and services that will help you to keep your dog fit and healthy. Almost all vet centres will be able to vaccinate your dog (see page 85). A good centre should also stock a range of healthcare products, including those designed for dental care and parasite control, and may stock special prepared diets to help in the treatment of specific conditions (see page 104).

Supplying you with products is, however, only a part of ensuring good healthcare for your dog. Even

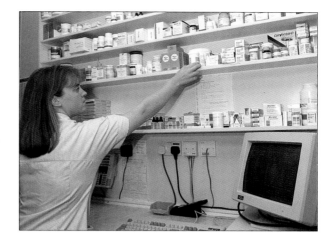

Vet centres stock a wide range of medicines for use on their patients. If you are given medicines for your dog, make sure that you know exactly when and how to administer them.

more important is the advice that you will need to select the most appropriate products and to use them properly. Your vet – or a nurse specially trained in all aspects of dog healthcare, including nutrition and dog behaviour – will give you invaluable advice. These nurses may offer advice on a one-to-one basis, but often run group clinics as well. 'Puppy parties' (see page 89) and slimming clinics are both examples.

REFERRALS

Very few vet centres have the necessary equipment and expertise to provide you with all the veterinary and healthcare services that your dog may need in his lifetime. If he requires procedures that are not available at your centre, your vet may suggest that you take him to see another vet, either at another vet centre or at a special referral hospital.

If necessary, your vet should also be able to refer you to other professionals who are involved in the care of animals, such as an animal-behaviour expert (see above, left) or even a physiotherapist, and should be able to make all the arrangements for you.

COMPLEMENTARY-THERAPY SERVICES

Complementary-therapy services are now becoming more commonly available through vet centres, and include homoeopathy, acupuncture and herbalism. If you would prefer your dog to be treated in this way whenever possible and appropriate, make sure that your vet centre understands your wishes in advance.

SURGICAL FEES

The fee for a surgical procedure carried out on your dog will consist of the cost of the anaesthetics, the operating-theatre time required and the cost of any other items used for the operation, such as cotton wool, syringes, needles and dressings. Remember that the technical skill of the surgeon and the equipment required are very advanced, and that you must expect a realistic bill.

Anaesthesia

Most dogs will experience a general anaesthetic at some point in their lives, but to many owners the thought of their dogs being anaesthetized and then submitted to an operation is a cause of great concern, often due to a fear of the unknown.

The following step-by-step outline of the events that are likely to take place if your dog needs a general anaesthetic should help to put your mind at rest. You should note, however, that the precise procedures may vary, depending both on the reason for your dog's anaesthetic and on the specific practices of the staff at your particular vet centre.

WHAT ARE ANAESTHETICS?

Anaesthetics allow a vet to carry out a diagnostic or surgical procedure safely and without causing pain. Two types of anaesthetic procedure are used on dogs.

LOCAL ANALGESIA
Special drugs may be used as injections, sprays, creams, gels or ointments to take away the sensation of pain from a specific part of the body. Surgical procedures carried out under local analgesia may include removing foreign bodies from the skin and treating small wounds.

GENERAL ANAESTHESIA
Anaesthetic drugs in the form of injectable liquids or breathable gases are used to intoxicate a dog's central nervous system. These cause loss of consciousness, prevent the awareness of pain and limit or relax the skeletal muscles, such as those of the limbs.

While a dog is under a general anaesthetic, his pulse and breathing rate will be constantly monitored.

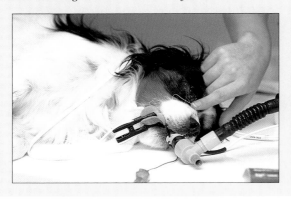

The night before the anaesthetic

You will normally be asked to withhold food from your dog after his dinner on the evening prior to the day of his anaesthetic. This is to make sure that he has an empty stomach when he is anaesthetized, as some drugs may stimulate him to vomit. You should not need to restrict his access to water in any way.

Admission

You will normally be asked to bring your dog to the vet centre first thing in the morning on the day of his operation. You should expect to be asked to sign a consent form, giving your authority for your dog to undergo certain specified procedures. Make sure that you read this form thoroughly.

Examination and pre-medication

Your dog will be examined by your vet or a veterinary nurse to check that there is nothing unexpected wrong with him. You will be asked to confirm that he has not eaten since the night before.

Your vet or nurse will then give your dog one or more injections – often referred to as the 'pre-med'. This is likely to include a tranquillizer or sedative drug that will help to relieve any anxiety, and will reduce the amount of general anaesthetic required later on.

You may be reluctant to leave your dog, but he may adjust to the situation more quickly if you disappear without too much fuss. Although many vet centres are happy for owners to stay with their dogs while the pre-med is administered, you may be encouraged to leave your dog before it is given.

The anaesthetic

As soon as the pre-med has taken effect and your vet is ready, your dog will be moved to a preparation room. Sitting or lying on a table, he will have an area of fur clipped from one foreleg, close to his elbow. This will be the place where the first part of the anaesthetic will be injected into a blood vessel called the cephalic vein.

Within seconds of the liquid anaesthetic entering the vein, your dog's legs will weaken and he will be helped to a lying position on his side. He will already be completely unconscious. Your vet will then pass a breathing pipe, called an endotracheal tube, down his windpipe, and the end of the tube will be connected to an anaesthetic machine. From this point onwards,

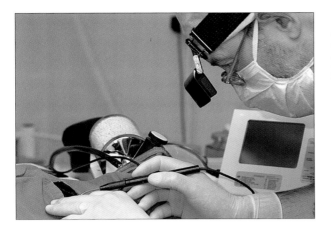

With the aid of modern equipment and advanced anaesthetic drugs, vets are able to carry out major surgical procedures that would not even have been attempted in the past.

your dog will be breathing a mixture of one or more anaesthetic gases and oxygen. His breathing and heart-rate, and his degree of unconsciousness, will be constantly monitored by the veterinary nurse.

Preparation

If your dog is to undergo surgery, the area of his body in which an incision is to be made will be clipped, and the skin will be cleaned with antibacterial solution. Your dog will then be moved to the operating theatre, where the cleaning will be repeated.

Meanwhile, your vet and any other assistants will be preparing themselves by scrubbing their hands with antibacterial soap and putting on sterile gowns, hats and gloves. Before beginning the operation, your vet will cover your dog's body – except the area in which the incision will be made – with sterile drapes.

The operation or procedure

Your vet will carry out the operation or procedure as quickly as is both safe and feasible, so that your dog is kept anaesthetized for the shortest time possible.

Recovery

The level of the anaesthetic will be reduced when your vet is close to finishing the surgery. Your dog will be disconnected from the anaesthetic machine, and will be taken to a recovery ward where he will be kept warm and comfortable while he wakes up. A nurse may administer further drugs such as painkillers or antibiotics, and will monitor his condition very closely.

The speed at which your dog wakes up will depend on his age and state of health, and on the anaesthetics used. If he is a young dog and has undergone a routine procedure, he may well regain consciousness within minutes and may be sitting up in half an hour.

Discharge from the vet centre

Most dogs anaesthetized for routine procedures go home the same day. Your vet or a nurse will give you specific advice regarding his nursing, and will tell you when they would like to see him again. Before leaving, make sure that you fully understand how and when to administer any medicines. Your dog should be able to walk, although he may be a little drowsy. You may be surprised at how bright he is, but he will still need special care (see below and pages 98–111).

At home

When you get home, take your dog to his bed and encourage him to rest. Use a wrapped hot-water bottle or other heat source to keep him warm (see page 106). Unless you have been advised otherwise, offer him a small meal if he appears interested in food: this may help him to sleep. Ensure that water is close to his bed, and encourage him to drink. Then leave him to rest.

Keep your dog quiet for the next few days, and strictly follow the advice that your vet has given you about his exercise and general management.

Before any procedure is carried out on your dog, make sure that you fully understand what will be done, and why.

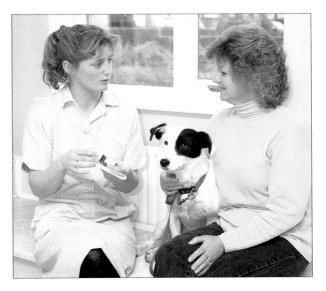

Special care

There are times when your dog will require very special care, such as when he is ill or recovering from an operation, or when he is simply growing old. For however long he needs it, his special care will become one of your main priorities: he will appreciate your time, as well as your love and concern.

Handling and restraining your dog

The type of care that your dog may need will depend on his condition, or on the procedure that he has undergone at your vet centre. Your vet, or a veterinary nurse, should tell you exactly what needs doing, and when and how to do it. Your responsibilities may involve carrying out any or all of the following tasks:
• Administering any medicines prescribed by your vet (see pages 101–3).
• Attending to any special dietary needs that your dog may have (see pages 104–5).
• Attending to his comfort and personal-hygiene needs (see pages 106–7).
• Adjusting your dog's lifestyle (see page 107).
• Attending to the care of any wounds and dressings (see pages 108–9).
• Monitoring your dog's progress and reporting back to your vet (see pages 110–11).

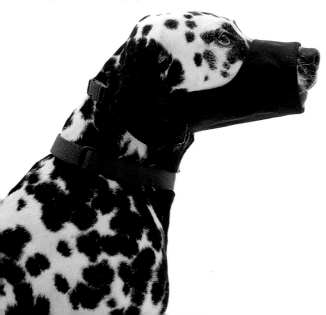

HANDLING TECHNIQUES

Whenever you carry out a physical examination or other procedure on your dog, it is essential that you handle him appropriately. By adopting the correct technique in a given situation, you should be able to carry out an examination or a nursing task quickly and effectively, without putting your safety at risk.

Your dog may not appreciate what you have to do to him, but a well-practised, slick approach will ensure that any discomfort that he may experience lasts for as short a time as is possible.

The following are some of the most important techniques for handling a dog.

Muzzling your dog

Even the most placid and normally well-behaved dog may bite as an instinctive reaction to pain or discomfort. It is much better to be safe than sorry, so always muzzle your dog before carrying out any kind of physical examination or medical procedure.

Several different types of muzzle are currently available for use on dogs. A plastic, 'basket'-style muzzle with an enclosed end is perhaps the safest of these. A fabric 'sleeve'-style muzzle (see left) is a good alternative, although some dogs may be able to nibble through the open end.

Whatever kind of muzzle you use, make sure that it is the correct size and shape for your dog. In an emergency situation, it is possible to make an effective makeshift muzzle using a length of cord, a scarf or any other suitable strong material (see opposite, above).

Sleeve-style muzzles are simple to use, comfortable for dogs to wear and easy to clean. They come in a number of sizes and are suitable for dogs with normal or long muzzles.

Tying a makeshift muzzle

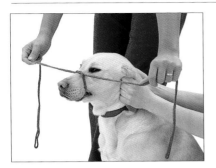

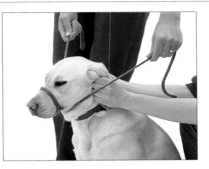

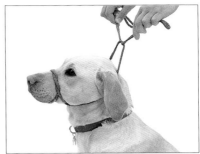

1 If you have an assistant, ask him or her to restrain your dog as shown. Make a loop in the cord and slip it over your dog's muzzle. Pull the knot firmly on top of his nose.

2 Pass the two ends of the cord underneath your dog's chin, cross them over, then bring them towards the back of his neck (take care not to pull the cord too tightly).

3 Pass the cord under your dog's ears. Finally, tie it in a secure knot – again, making sure that you do not pull the cord too tightly – at the back of his head.

Lifting your dog

You should take great care not to cause yourself – or your dog – any injury when you lift him up, especially if he is large or heavy. Adopting the following lifting techniques should prevent either of you from coming to any harm.

On your own • Place one arm under your dog's neck and grasp the elbow that is furthest away from you. Scoop up his bottom with your other arm, holding on to his knee as you do so.

With assistance • Position one arm under your dog's chest, and the other under his neck. Ask your helper to support your dog's rear end, and then lift him up in one co-ordinated movement.

(Note that, depending on your dog's condition, you may need to adapt these techniques to avoid putting pressure on any injuries or wounds that he may have.)

Carrying your dog

Before carrying your dog from one place to another, make sure that your path is clear and that all doors are open. You can carry a small- or medium-sized dog by supporting his rear end on one arm and embracing him around his chest with the other. A large dog will be best carried using the lifting technique described above.

A dog who is used to being picked up and carried from a young age will be easier to handle as an adult. Do not attempt to lift your dog unless you are sure that you can manage his weight.

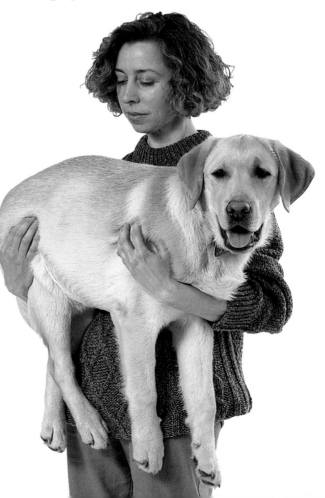

RESTRAINT TECHNIQUES

Proper restraint will be especially important when your dog is ill or injured, because his behaviour may become unpredictable if he feels uncomfortable or is in pain. Even if your dog is the most gentle of souls under normal circumstances, you simply cannot tell how he will react in such a situation, so you must always err on the side of safety.

In order to carry out some nursing procedures on your dog – such as changing a bandage or a dressing on a skin wound – you will need someone to assist you. One of you will then be able to restrain your dog and reassure him if he becomes at all anxious, while the other concentrates on carrying out the procedure as quickly and smoothly as possible.

Restraining your dog while standing

Place one arm around your dog's neck, and the other under his stomach to prevent him from sitting down. Your hold on his neck should be sufficiently firm that it is impossible for him either to turn his head to the side, or to lunge forwards.

Restraining your dog while sitting

Place one arm around your dog's neck (as above), and then place your other arm over his back and under his chest. Use the forearm and elbow of this arm to keep your dog's body tucked closely into yours.

HANDLING TIPS

• Avoid trying to restrain your dog on the ground, unless he is too heavy for you to lift, or his condition makes this inappropriate. An old table covered with a non-slip mat makes an ideal examination and treatment bench.
• Always try to match the degree of restraint to the procedure that you wish to carry out. The general rule of animal nursing is to use the minimum restraint that is necessary to ensure both effective and safe control.
• Be firm but kind, and sensitive to your dog's mood. If you are not sufficiently firm and your dog feels insecure, he may try to escape; if you are too firm, he may panic.
• Give your dog clear commands, such as 'SIT', 'LIE' or 'STAY'. Tell him what you are doing, as he will find your voice reassuring.

You should practise restraining your dog when he is a puppy, to make him easier to handle as an adult dog.

Restraining your dog in a lying position

In order to carry out some medical procedures on your dog – such as the application of an ointment or cream to his skin – you may need to restrain him in a lying position.

As with the methods of restraint described above, you should ideally have an assistant, especially if your dog is large and strong. However, if he is easy to handle you should be able to manage on your own.

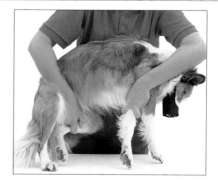

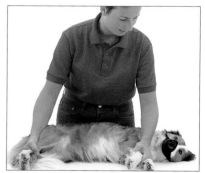

1 With your dog standing (ideally, on a suitable table), lean over him and grasp the foreleg that is nearest to you with one hand, and the hindleg on the same side with the other. Slowly but firmly, lift these legs off the table. Your dog will start to lean against you. As he does so, move his legs away from your body. He should then start to slide down your front, and will end up lying on his side.

2 Adjust your hold to rest the forearm that is restraining your dog's foreleg over his neck, in order to keep his head on the table. Move your other arm over his bottom to prevent him from trying to sit up.

Administering medicines

Most ill dogs will be treated as out-patients of vet centres, so your vet is likely to ask you to give medicines to your dog at home when he is unwell. In addition, even when your dog is healthy you will need to medicate him regularly against common conditions such as intestinal-worm infestations (see pages 32–4).

Always read the instructions on any medication very carefully, and follow strictly the recommendations that you are given by your vet or a veterinary nurse. He or she should be happy to give you a demonstration if you are unsure about a particular technique.

If you do not feel confident about administering a medicine to your dog, say so. Your vet may be able to prescribe a treatment that is designed to be given in a different way, or may even arrange for your dog to have his medication administered at your vet centre as and when necessary (in the latter case, he may need to be treated as an in-patient).

Safety first

Unless your dog is very calm, and is well-accustomed to health-checks and oral examinations, always try to arrange for someone else to help you handle him when administering medicines (see pages 98–100). Another pair of hands will make the task less stressful for you and your dog, and you will be more likely to succeed in administering the medicine at the first attempt.

Avoid medicating your dog on the ground or on your lap: you are much more likely to keep control of him if he is on a table with a non-slip surface.

Giving tablets and capsules

Tablets and capsules are generally given by mouth. Most dogs will tolerate being force-fed with medicines in this way, and some of them actively seem to enjoy the experience, obviously believing that a palatable tablet or capsule is an unusual – but nevertheless a very welcome – treat!

Before you begin, check the dose on the medicine label. If you are in any doubt, contact your vet centre for advice before going further.

USEFUL TIPS

• Coat tablets with butter to help them to slip down.
• The further you tilt your dog's head back, the less tension there will be in his jaw and the easier it will be to drop a tablet or capsule on to the back of his tongue.
• Do not crush tablets or open capsules without first checking with your vet that this will not affect them.

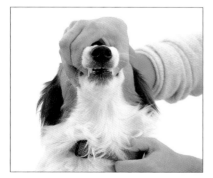

1 Place the palm of your hand on your dog's muzzle, with your thumb and index finger on either side of it. Keeping a firm grip, rotate your wrist to turn his face upwards. His lower jaw should start to open.

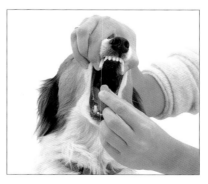

2 Holding the tablet or capsule in your free hand, use your middle finger to open your dog's mouth by pulling down on his teeth. Drop the tablet or capsule into the back of his mouth, and then quickly close it.

3 Keep your dog looking skyward by supporting his chin, and gently rub down his throat to encourage him to swallow.

Giving liquid medicines, syrups and emulsions

Check the dose on the container, and shake the contents if specified. Draw up the medicine into the supplied dropper or syringe.

Support your dog's head firmly with one hand around his muzzle, and tip his head back slightly. Place the end of the dropper or syringe into his mouth, behind his canine, or 'eye' tooth. Aiming across his mouth rather than down his throat, gently administer the medicine.

If your dog chews at the dropper or syringe, do not worry as this will actually encourage him to swallow. If he begins to cough, immediately lower his head. When he has settled down, try again more slowly.

Administering ear drops and ointment

Muzzle your dog, then gently clean away any discharge from around his ear hole and on the inner side of his ear flap, using cotton wool wetted with plain water or with a special ear-cleaning solution.

Check the dose on the medicine container, and shake ear drops if this is specified.

It may be difficult for you to tell how many drops or how much of the ointment you are administering. It is therefore a very good idea to practise first in a kitchen sink, in order to find out how hard you will need to squeeze the tube or bottle to deliver the correct quantity of medicine into your dog's ear.

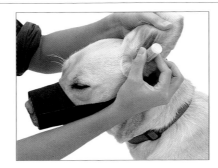

1 Take the base of your dog's ear flap between the thumb and index finger of one hand. Hold the medicine-container nozzle in the other, just above the ear hole, and administer the drops or ointment.

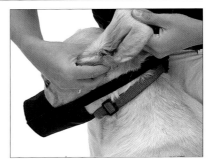

2 Your dog will shake his head, but do not let go of his ear flap until you have massaged the skin and underlying cartilage. This will encourage the drops or ointment to flow down towards his ear drum.

Administering eye drops

Muzzle your dog, then gently wipe away any discharge from around his eye or eyes, using cotton wool wetted with plain water or with a special eye-bath solution that has been recommended by your vet.

Check the dose on the container, and shake the contents thoroughly if this is specified.

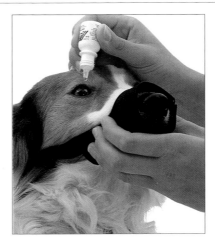

1 Hold the bottle between the thumb and index finger of one hand, and use your other hand to support your dog's head firmly, by cupping it under his muzzle. Tip his head back slightly, and use your free fingers to apply tension to his eyelids to prevent him from blinking for a second or two.

Hold the dropper bottle a short distance away from your dog's eye, and squeeze the required number of drops directly on to his eyeball. Be very careful to avoid holding the bottle too close when you do this as, if your dog moves suddenly, you could poke his eye with it.

2 Release your dog's head and allow him to blink. His eyelids will disperse the medicine over the surface of his eyeball.

Administering eye ointment

Muzzle your dog, then clean away any discharge from his eye. Check the dose on the container.

1 Gently pull back your dog's upper and lower eyelids to keep them apart. Holding the tube parallel to the lower eyelid, squeeze out the ointment so that it falls on to the edge of the lower eyelid.

2 Release your dog's head and allow him to blink once or twice. Then carefully massage his upper and lower eyelids together, as this will help to smear the ointment over the surface of the eyeball.

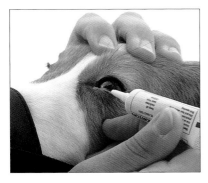

FURTHER TIPS ON GIVING MEDICINES

TOPICAL TREATMENTS
Shampoos, ointments, creams, sprays, liquid drops, powders and foams are all used to treat skin conditions, and are generally straightforward to apply.

In order to prevent your dog from licking off any medication applied to his skin, you may need to fit him with an 'Elizabethan collar' (see page 108). Another useful trick is to apply the medication just before feeding your dog, so that he is otherwise occupied while it begins to take effect.

MEDICINES IN FOOD
Some – but not all – medicines may be mixed with a dog's food to make administration easier. However, dogs have a keen sense of smell and are usually extremely good at detecting 'doctored' food. For this reason, it is best to choose a very smelly, moist food that your dog enjoys. Heat the food to body temperature before mixing in the medicine: this will help to release pleasant odours and to disguise the odour of the medication.

CONSULTING YOUR VET
Never administer drugs intended for human use – including painkillers – to your dog without consulting your vet.

FINISH THE COURSE
Always complete the administration of a course of medication prescribed for your dog by your vet. Do not miss a dose, and do not stop treatment just because you think that his symptoms have improved. Many treatment courses are designed to be continued for a few days after apparent recovery and, if you stop the medication too early, your dog's illness may well recur.

IF YOU HAVE PROBLEMS
If you experience any difficulty in medicating your dog, or if he appears to react badly to being medicated, contact your vet centre immediately.

If you are unsure of any technique, ask your vet for a demonstration.

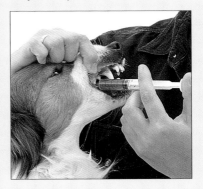

Food and drink

If feeding a specific diet is appropriate to your dog's condition, your vet will advise you accordingly. It is likely that he or she will recommend basing your dog's diet while he is ill on a prepared food proven to help in the treatment of his condition (see below, right).

Dietary adjustments feature prominently in the treatment regimes for a number of major conditions, including the following:
• Dogs with certain types of diarrhoea (see pages 30–1) benefit from highly digestible, low-fat, low-fibre meals.
• Dogs with chronic renal failure (see page 67) may benefit from a diet containing restricted amounts of protein, phosphorus and sodium.
• Dogs with urolithiasis (see page 69) may be treated by feeding a diet that has a direct effect on their urine and dissolves the uroliths.
• Obese dogs (see pages 82–3) need foods with reduced calorie contents to help them to lose weight.
• Old dogs often benefit from reduced-calorie diets that contain less protein, phosphorus and sodium, and higher levels of certain vitamins, fatty acids and zinc.

SPECIAL NUTRITIONAL NEEDS

A short period of under-eating in a healthy dog will not cause severe problems, but under-nourishment in a dog whose body is stressed by disease, injury or surgery is likely to have much more serious consequences. Such a dog may be prone to the following problems:
• A decrease in his liver and muscle energy stores, forcing him to burn off his own tissues to provide his body with fuel (even after minor surgery, a dog may use 10 per cent more fuel each day; if he suffers a severe burn, his energy requirement may increase much more.
• Adverse effects on the immune system, leading to increased susceptibility to infections.
• Muscle wastage
• Shock
• Delayed healing of wounds

Avoiding under-nourishment

If your dog has not eaten normal amounts of food for three to five days as a result of illness, injury or surgery, or is suffering from muscle wastage due to illness, your vet may recommend a diet with the following elements:
• Fat as the main source of energy
• Sufficient protein to support normal growth
• Sufficient vitamins, minerals and essential fatty acids to support normal growth .
• Increased amounts of zinc

Convalescent diets

Special diets have now been formulated to meet the nutritional needs of stressed dogs who have reduced appetites, and should be available from your vet centre. These are highly palatable, and are made in a liquid form that can be administered by syringe if necessary.

As these diets are very concentrated and are high in calories, only small volumes are needed to supply an ill dog's needs. A dog's daily food allocation is normally best split into five or six small meals.

Administering solid food using a syringe

1 Ask your vet for a suitable-sized syringe, and cut off the end. Pull out the plunger and then push the cut-off syringe into the food so that you scoop a core of food into it.

2 Hold the syringe close to your dog's nose so that he can smell the food. As he opens his mouth, insert the syringe and gently push the plunger to deliver the food on to his tongue. If your dog will not open his mouth, you may need to do this (see page 103, bottom right).

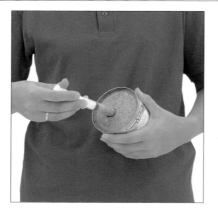

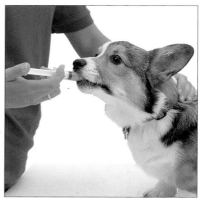

FEEDING AN ILL DOG

Ensuring that a dog who is reluctant to eat receives adequate nourishment takes patience. Offering highly palatable, warmed food, or smearing small amounts of food on his lips may encourage a dog to eat.

Forced feeding

A dog who will not eat voluntarily must be force-fed. The most common methods are as follows:
• Placing small lumps of food on the back of the dog's tongue and encouraging him to swallow. The technique is similar to that used to administer tablets and capsules by mouth (see page 101).
• Administering solid food by syringe (see below, left).
• Administering liquid food by syringe (see right). However, forced feeding may cause some dogs further stress. Such dogs may be fitted with feeding tubes to deliver liquid food directly into their digestive systems.

FLUIDS

A dog can survive for weeks without food, but he will only remain alive for a few days without water. He will constantly lose water from his body in his faeces and urine, in the air that he breathes out, in the small amount of sweat that he produces through his feet and nose, and in his other body secretions.

All this lost water must be replaced. Some will be produced by the dog's body as it burns food to produce energy, and some will be contained in his food, but the rest must come from drinking.

Fluids for a healthy dog

A labrador retriever's body contains about 18 litres (4 gallons) of water, accounting for 60 per cent of his body weight. A dog of this type will need a minimum of about 1.5 litres (2½ pints) of water per day, obtained from eating and drinking. It is impossible to know how much water your dog will lose each day, so he should always have access to fresh water: he can then adjust his intake to suit himself.

Fluids for an ill dog

A dog's fluid requirements when he is ill will depend on his condition. If the labrador retriever previously mentioned were to suffer from a fever, he could double his fluid requirements; if he has severe diarrhoea, he will lose much more fluid than usual in his faeces. Even if he is just not eating normally, he will need to drink more to compensate for the decrease in his water intake.

When your dog is recovering from illness, your vet is likely to ask you to monitor his water intake. He or she will then advise you whether you need to give him fluids by mouth to prevent dehydration (see below). However, as with food, forcing your dog to drink may distress him, in which case your vet may put him on a drip (see page 95) to replace any shortfall of fluids.

Special fluids

Depending on your dog's condition, your vet may advise giving him a special fluid instead of plain water. For instance, if your dog has had diarrhoea, he should recover more quickly if given water containing certain chemicals. These are available as prepared powders, or you can make up a solution of 5 ml (1 teaspoonful) of salt and 10 ml (1 dessertspoonful) of glucose to 2 litres (3½ pints) of water.

To administer water or liquidized food, tilt up your dog's head, place the tip of the syringe in his mouth and gently empty the contents.

Environment and personal hygiene

Offering your dog a quiet, peaceful and warm place to rest will help his convalescence. Your vet or a veterinary nurse will give you specific advice on your dog's basic management during this period.

Recovery from routine surgery is normally very straightforward, and your main management priority may be to control your dog's activity. However, if he has been seriously ill or has undergone major surgery, his management is likely to be much more complex: it may then involve caring for his personal-hygiene needs and even taking on the role of his physiotherapist.

The following are some of the management issues relating to the nursing care of a convalescing dog that may be appropriate to your dog's condition.

Your dog's bed

This should be in a secluded place, but where you can easily keep an eye on him. His immediate environment should be quiet and warm, with a low lighting level.

Your dog's bedding should be warm, soft and easily washable. The bedding that is used in most vet centres is a type of man-made fleece, which can be washed in a conventional washing machine and dries rapidly.

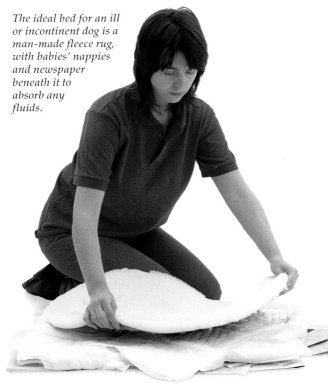

The ideal bed for an ill or incontinent dog is a man-made fleece rug, with babies' nappies and newspaper beneath it to absorb any fluids.

PROVIDING WARMTH

You can keep your dog warm in a number of ways, without making his environment stuffy.
• Electric heated pads are available that are designed to be placed under a dog's bedding.
• You can place a hot-water bottle in his bed (this must be covered and not placed in contact with his skin).
• You can place blankets over your dog.

Confinement

Your vet may tell you that your dog's activity must be restricted to lying down, sitting, standing and turning around. This can be achieved using a dog crate (look in dog magazines for specialist suppliers), or by fencing off an area with boarding or other appropriate material.

No matter how confined your dog has to be, he should still be able to move around enough to find a comfortable position to lie in. Some hyperactive dogs require short-term sedation during their convalescence.

Hair care

If your dog has long hair, you must keep it clean and well-groomed. If it remains soiled or becomes matted, he may suffer skin problems that could complicate his condition. Grooming may also have a therapeutic effect.

If your dog is incontinent, it may be sensible to trim away any long hair from under his tail, while smearing some petroleum jelly on the hair around a male dog's penis or a bitch's vulva will help to prevent urine-scalding of the skin. Despite taking these measures, you may still need to bathe parts of your dog regularly.

Claw care

If your dog has a long convalescence and is not able to exercise normally, his claws may become overgrown. If so, ask your vet or a veterinary nurse to cut them for him, or carefully trim them yourself (see pages 64–5).

Personal hygiene

If your dog has a dry mouth, you can moisten it for him by gently wiping his gums with a damp sponge, squeezing out a little water as you do so. He must be awake when you do this, so that he can swallow any excess water. Regularly and frequently wipe away any accumulated discharge around his nose, eyes or mouth using moist face-wipes.

Cleaning your dog's bottom

1 When your dog is ill, he may well soil the area under his tail. To keep his bottom as clean and hygienic as possible, ask someone to restrain him and then carefully trim the hair using curved scissors. Wash away the worst of any soiling using warm water and cotton wool.

2 Finish off by gently wiping the area using wet wipes. Once you have cut your dog's hair short, you should be able to keep his bottom clean simply by using the wipes.

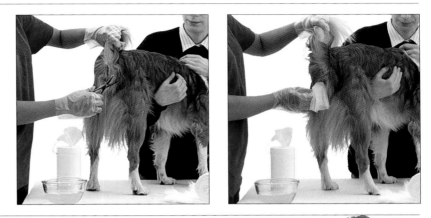

Mental and physical stimulation

Your dog will welcome the reassurance of your touch and your voice, so spend time stroking and talking to him. Do not let him lie in one position for too long: if he cannot move himself, gently turn him every few hours.

If your dog is alert but must be confined, give him toys to keep him stimulated. A hollow toy stuffed with a little tasty food may keep him amused for hours.

If your dog can walk, you should regularly take him outside to enjoy some fresh air. Make sure that you keep control of him by putting on his lead if necessary.

Physiotherapy

By gently manipulating your dog's joints, you will help to prevent the stiffness caused by inactivity. If he has had orthopaedic (bone) surgery, your vet may ask you to carry out specific physiotherapy techniques.

Exercise

If your dog is recovering from routine surgery, your vet may advise you to restrict him to lead-walking until his wound has healed and his stitches have been removed.

Your dog's condition may mean altering his exercise regime for good. For instance, a dog with arthritis (see pages 46–7) may benefit from frequent, short bouts of restrained activity – even swimming, in warm weather.

Toileting

If your dog is at all mobile, you should encourage him to go to the toilet regularly, particularly when he wakes up from sleeping and after eating. If he can sit up, but is too weak or disabled to use his hindlegs properly,

you can support his rear end using a towel slung under his abdomen (see below), or a special harness.

If your dog cannot move, he will have to urinate and defecate where he lies. Clean up after him regularly, and place towels or babies' nappies beneath his bedding to soak up the urine and keep him dry.

If your dog cannot support his own weight on his hindlegs, you can help him by using a towel as a sling (you must check first with your vet that he or she is happy for you to use this technique).

Wound management

If your dog is recovering from a traumatic or surgical wound, or an uncomfortable skin condition, it is important that he does not damage the affected area further or interfere with the normal healing process through licking, biting, or scratching.

PROTECTING A WOUND
The method that your vet will recommend to prevent self-trauma will depend on the nature of your dog's wound or skin condition, the degree of irritation that it is causing, the part of the body affected, your dog's temperament and your availability to supervise him. The following are all commonly employed options.

Wound coverings
A range of dressings, bandages (see opposite, below) and other coverings, including rigid casts, may be used to protect and stabilize wounds.

'Elizabethan collars'
These are effective devices for preventing self-trauma through licking and biting. If your dog needs to wear this type of collar, only remove it when you can watch over him.

Often known as 'lampshades', Elizabethan collars are a simple but effective way of preventing dogs from nibbling at themselves. They are available in a range of sizes: your vet or a nurse will select the correct one for your dog.

'Anti-chew' preparations
These supposedly foul-tasting concoctions are applied to a dog's skin to discourage him from licking and chewing it. They do appear to work with some dogs, but others seem to like the taste or totally ignore it!

Muzzles
Putting a basket-type muzzle on your dog (see page 98) will prevent him from licking or chewing at a wound or dressing. However, a dog wearing this type of muzzle may use the edges to scratch at the area, and can cause a surprising amount of damage in a short time.

Distraction
If your dog is well-behaved, you should be able to discourage him from interfering with a wound by means of discipline and distraction. As soon as he shows any interest in his wound, say 'NO' in a clear and stern voice in order to break his concentration, and then immediately offer him an alternative source of entertainment such as a hollow toy with a small amount of his favourite food hidden inside it.

Sedation
Some dogs are so hyperactive that short-term sedation during recovery is the only way to force them to rest and to leave any wounds alone.

DRESSINGS, BANDAGES AND CASTS
These may be used to protect a wound from further injury, infection or self-trauma, to immobilize a bone fracture (see pages 48–9), dislocation or joint sprain, or to apply pressure to stop bleeding or control swelling.

The care of any dressings, bandages or casts will involve the following:
• Protecting them from becoming wet, soiled or otherwise damaged: bandages and casts should be covered by a plastic bag or a proprietary waterproof sock when exposed to wet conditions.

WARNING
Take great care not to apply a bandage or adhesive tape too tightly around one of your dog's legs. Doing so may adversely affect the blood supply to the wound, as well as to the part of the body below the bandage.

• Preventing your dog from damaging or even removing them himself: all the techniques detailed opposite for protecting wounds are appropriate.

• Removing and replacing them: this will normally be carried out at your vet centre, but you may be asked to change a simple dressing in order to bathe a wound that requires frequent cleaning.

Changing a bandage or dressing

Before attempting to change a bandage or dressing on your dog, make sure that your vet or a veterinary nurse has given you any products – such as antibacterial solutions, creams, dressings and bandages – that you will need, as well as precise instructions and a practical demonstration of what to do.

The procedure that your vet is likely to ask you to carry out is as follows:

1 Muzzle your dog for safety, and then ask an assistant to restrain him properly for you on a suitable surface (such as a table covered with a non-slip mat).

2 Remove the existing bandage by unwrapping it (do not use scissors to cut it off, as you could injure your dog if he were to move suddenly).

3 Carefully unwrap any underlying padding and peel off any dressing. If either the padding or the dressing has stuck to the wound, moisten any adhered areas with warm water to loosen them.

4 Gently bathe the wound or affected area of skin before re-dressing it, following the instructions of your vet or veterinary nurse.

Bandaging a paw

One of the most common types of wound coverings is a paw bandage, and the very vulnerable location of such bandages means that they often require frequent changing when they become damaged or wet.

If your dog damages a claw (see pages 64–5) or cuts a paw, you may need to bandage it as a first-aid procedure, to protect the injury and to make your dog more comfortable before taking him to your vet. The bandaging technique outlined here can also be adapted to the covering of other leg wounds.

To prepare the wound ready for bandaging, you should clean it thoroughly by placing your dog's paw in a bowl of warm, salty water or veterinary antiseptic solution. Keep changing the cleaning solution if it becomes dirty. If the wound starts to bleed, you should move on to dressing and bandaging it straight away.

Gently dry off the paw as well as you can, using a clean towel. If the wound is bleeding or moist, cover it with a piece of impregnated gauze (see page 115).

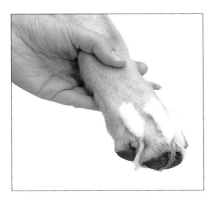

1 Fill the gaps between each of your dog's toes with a small wad of cotton wool. Then wrap the paw with cotton wool peeled from a roll, to a thickness of 2 cm (¾ in).

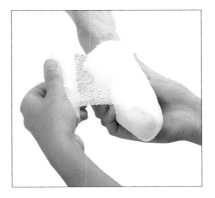

2 To compress the cotton wool, apply an open-weave bandage backwards and forwards over the toes and around the paw, leaving a ring of cotton wool at the top.

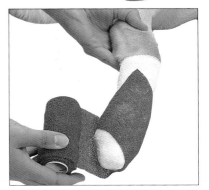

3 Wrap an adhesive bandage over the top. Secure the end with medical adhesive tape, wrapping this loosely around the top so that it sticks to the bandage and to the fur.

Monitoring an ill dog

By diligently monitoring your dog's condition, you will quickly notice if he is not progressing as he should do. The nature and degree of monitoring needed will depend on the seriousness of his illness or injury.

Before you bring your dog home from your vet centre after medical treatment or a surgical procedure, be sure to find out what monitoring procedures you should undertake. Ask what – if any – specific signs you should look out for in your dog's appearance, as well as in his behaviour and inputs and outputs (see opposite).

The following monitoring procedures are commonly carried out by veterinary nurses on their in-patients, and will be relevant to your nursing care at home.

Physical examinations

Carry out an examination of your dog's anatomy once a day (see pages 8–9). Any abnormal features of his appearance – including the following – may represent cause for concern:

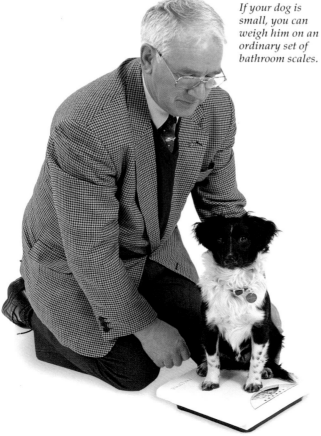

If your dog is small, you can weigh him on an ordinary set of bathroom scales.

While your dog is convalescing, measure how much water he drinks each day. In the morning, fill his bowl to a set level. Over the next 24 hours, record how much you need to add to keep it at this level: the total will be the amount that your dog has drunk.

• Dull, sunken or staring eyes
• Pale, dry gums
• The sudden appearance on his bedding or coat of blood or other discharges.
• An unexpected swelling associated with a wound
• An abnormal or foul smell associated with a wound, bandage or cast, with his body as a whole, or with his environment in general.

Weighing

A decrease in your dog's weight during convalescence may be due to inadequate feeding or to dehydration (see pages 104–5), so regular and frequent weighing is an essential monitoring procedure. You should weigh your dog at the same time each day if at all possible.

Behaviour monitoring

Obvious signs of discomfort include the following:
• Sudden lethargy, dullness or reluctance to move
• Panting
• Lack of tail-wagging and interest in the presence of familiar people.
• Crying, howling or barking
• Sudden mood changes
• Aggression when handled
• Restlessness

Inputs: food and water

When your dog is convalescing from an illness, injury or surgery, you will need to make adjustments to his dietary regime if he fails to eat normally for more than a day or two (see pages 104–5).

It will also be essential to monitor accurately his water intake, as any shortfalls must be replaced by other means, such as forced administration by mouth or directly into his bloodstream via an intravenous drip (see page 95).

Outputs: urine and faeces

By keeping an eye on the quantity and appearance of the urine produced by your convalescent dog each day you will be able to monitor his basic kidney function, while the nature and quantity of any faeces produced will give a good indication as to the condition of his digestive system. Your vet will advise you on what to look for when checking your dog's urine and faeces.

Body temperature

You may be asked to take your dog's temperature on a regular basis while he is convalescing, to identify the first signs of fever development. Most healthy dogs have a rectal temperature of about 39°C (102°F).

You should use the following technique to take your dog's temperature, with the help of an assistant to restrain him (see page 100):

1 Check that the thermometer is re-set to zero, cover its end with a lubricant jelly and then carefully insert it into the centre of your dog's anal ring by twisting

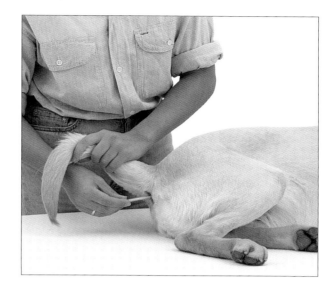

Your vet or a veterinary nurse will demonstrate how to take your dog's temperature, and will tell you how often to do so (in most cases, this will be twice a day).

the thermometer gently. Insert it sufficiently far that the tip is well through the anal ring.

2 Holding on to the thermometer throughout, leave it in place for 30 to 60 seconds (follow the instructions for use supplied with your thermometer).

3 Gently remove the thermometer and wipe it clean with cotton wool. Read the recorded temperature and write it down, along with the date and time.

PULSE AND RESPIRATION RATES

A dog's pulse is taken on his inner thigh, close to his groin. It can be fairly difficult to feel in some dogs. The pulse rate of a healthy dog at rest is normally 70–140 beats per minute.

Measure your dog's breathing rate by watching how many times his rib cage rises and falls in one minute. If this is difficult to see, gently pluck a small tuft of loose fur from his coat and hold it in front of his nostrils: it will move as he breathes in and out. The breathing rate of a healthy dog at rest is normally 10–30 breaths per minute.

If you are not confident about any monitoring procedure, ask your vet or a veterinary nurse for a demonstration.

Taking a dog's pulse is not as easy as it may at first appear. Practise taking your dog's pulse when he is healthy, so that you are experienced at doing so when a real need arises.

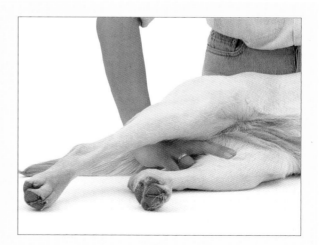

Preventive healthcare

If you are anything like me, you will never remember when you should be having your eyes tested or your tetanus vaccination updated, but now you have your dog's health to look after as well.

Some healthcare tasks – such as feeding – obviously need to be carried out daily, and not even I would need reminding to do that. However, other procedures such as vaccination and worming are required less frequently, and can easily be overlooked or delayed.

The information given here relates to a typical dog living in the UK and starts from the age of eight weeks, when many puppies move to their new homes. Use this, together with the specific advice of your vet, to create a customized healthcare plan for your dog.

ROUTINE HEALTH-CHECKS

Taking your dog for veterinary check-ups, and carrying out health-checks at home, are both very important aspects of preventive heathcare.

A puppy
With a vet • At eight weeks, 12 weeks and 12 months.
With a veterinary nurse • Physical-development and growth checks (ideally, every four weeks).
At home • Once a week, including weighing (see pages 8–9).

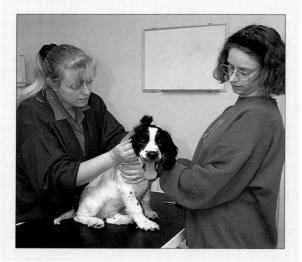

An adult dog
With a vet • Every 12 months.
At home • Once a week (see pages 8–9).

PARASITE CONTROL

Worming against parasitic intestinal tapeworms and roundworms (see pages 32–4), and treating your dog and house for fleas (see pages 58–9).

Tapeworms
First dose • At eight weeks.
Subsequent doses • Every two to three months.

Roundworms
First dose • At eight weeks.
Second dose • At 10 weeks.
Third dose • At 12 weeks.
Subsequent doses • Every three months.

Flea prevention
Your dog • This will vary, depending on the product used. A typical spray is designed to be used every two weeks.
Your house • Every four months: spraying with an appropriate insecticide.

DIETARY CHANGES

From puppy to adult food • At maturity (usually at six to 12 months, depending on the breed).

To food for an older dog • At five to seven years old, depending on the breed (see page 81).

TIMINGS OF TREATMENTS

The exact timing of certain procedures and events will vary depending on many factors, such as the nature of products used, the predicted parasite and worm burden in the area in which you live, and the prevailing views of the veterinary profession in your country.

Ask at your vet centre for more precise information relating to your particular dog.

VACCINATIONS

Initial course

Against distemper, canine parvovirus, canine leptospirosis and infectious canine hepatitis; canine parainfluenza virus may also be included (see pages 42–3 and 84–5).
First vaccination • At six to 10 weeks.
Second vaccination • At 12 weeks.

Booster vaccinations

Against canine parvovirus and canine leptospirosis; canine parainfluenza virus may also be included.
First booster • At 15 months.
Subsequent vaccinations • Every 12 months (distemper and infectious canine hepatitis are needed every other year, starting at 27 months).

Extra vaccination

Against *Bordetella* bacteria (see pages 42–3), four weeks prior to going to boarding kennels.

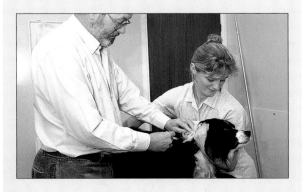

NEUTERING

A bitch • Ideally, before or after the first heat, or between subsequent heats (see pages 70–1).
A male dog • At about six months old, or at any time thereafter (see page 72).

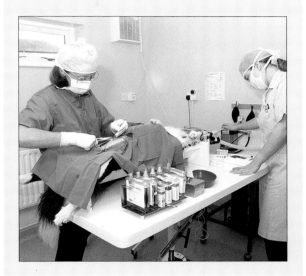

GROOMING

At home • A quick groom daily; a thorough groom once a week.
With a professional groomer • Every six months.

YOUR DOG'S DIARY

A record of your dog's individual anatomical quirks, together with other personal details, is a very valuable document. Keeping a special diary updated can also become a project that many children and adults will find both entertaining and educational.

This diary should include all your dog's identification details such as his size, eye colour and markings: this information may prove vital if he is lost. It should also specify all relevant care information, including examples of labels from his food.

Accidents and emergencies

This section of the book tells you how to cope with some of the most common accident-and-emergency situations in which your dog may be involved. You should familiarize yourself now with the contents of the information given here, so that in the event of an emergency you will be less likely to panic.

Coping with an emergency

If your dog suddenly becomes ill or is badly injured in some way, it is very important that you try to stay calm. His life may be quite literally in your hands until your vet or a veterinary nurse can take over from you.

The step-by-step guides on the following pages give practical directions relating to some of the most common emergency situations to affect dogs. Painful, but less critical, situations – such as lameness resulting from a thorn in your dog's paw – are covered in the relevant sections elsewhere in the book.

What constitutes an emergency?

Those situations that constitute emergencies will vary from owner to owner: for example, an event that may be considered an emergency by an inexperienced dog-owner may be less cause for concern to someone who has lived with dogs for years. However, some accidents and illnesses are obvious emergencies to all.

An emergency is any situation affecting your dog that you believe may be causing him undue pain or placing his life in danger. If you are at all unsure as to whether your dog needs urgent medical attention, it is much better to be over-cautious and to contact your vet centre for advice. Your vet or a veterinary nurse will be able to give you instructions over the telephone as to what actions to take, and, if you are worrying unnecessarily, will put your mind at rest.

What to do first

If your dog is injured, or suddenly shows what you interpret to be serious symptoms of illness, contact your vet centre as soon as you can. Only delay this in order to carry out resuscitation techniques (see pages 116–17) or to deal with an immediately life-threatening situation such as bleeding. Ideally, you should stay with your dog and carry out first aid while another person telephones for help.

The staff at your vet centre will give you specific instructions. If your dog can be moved, your vet is likely to suggest that you take him straight to the centre so that he can benefit from its facilities.

Dealing with a dog in pain

A dog's natural instinct when he is frightened, injured or in pain is to run away from whatever he thinks is causing the fear or the pain. As a result, many injured dogs may be shy and highly suspicious of people, including their owners.

For instance, it is not unusual for a dog who has a broken leg to disappear from the scene of an accident altogether. In such a situation, your natural instinct may be to chase after him and catch him so that you can help him. However, by running after him in this way – especially with other people – you are likely to drive him further away and frighten him even more. Instead, you should do the following:

BE PREPARED

- If you are unsure about how to perform any of the practical procedures covered in this section, ask your vet or a veterinary nurse for a demonstration.
- Where appropriate, practise the special handling techniques on your dog when he is fit and healthy, so that you will be able to carry them out both quickly and efficiently in a crisis situation.
- Take this book with you whenever you go away with your dog: you never know when you might have need of the information that it contains.

1 Call your dog's name to try to identify where he is.
2 Keep talking to him in a calm and friendly voice.
3 Organize any helpers to form a circle around him: this may discourage him from running away.
4 Make sure that you have your dog's lead or another method of keeping hold of him when you do get close to him, as well as something to make into an emergency muzzle, should he become aggressive (see page 99).
5 Get down to your dog's level, and keep talking to him. Only move closer to him when he seems calm, and, if he looks anxious and flighty, stop moving.
6 Your dog may let you stroke him and attach his lead, but if he is in pain he may resent you touching him at all. Wrap a piece of clothing around an arm to fend off an attack while attaching the lead.
7 Before carrying out any first aid, muzzle your dog or ask a helper to restrain him (see pages 98–100). Remember that even the most trustworthy dog may become aggressive when he is hurt.

EMERGENCY CHECKLIST

In any emergency situation, your priorities should be to do the following:
• Apprehend your dog if he is free (see left).
• Carry out any essential first-aid procedures to save your dog's life or to reduce his pain before he can receive veterinary attention (see pages 116–23).
• Contact your vet centre for advice, or to arrange for the assistance of your vet or a veterinary nurse.
• Keep your dog warm by wrapping him in a foil blanket or in a sheet of bubble-wrap if you have your first-aid kit with you (see below). If possible, you can also let him share your body heat.
• Keep your dog calm and quiet.
• Prevent him from suffering further injury. Unless it is imperative to move your dog for safety reasons, only move him if you are sure that it is safe to do so, or if you are advised to do so by veterinary staff.
• Prevent your dog from injuring you or anyone else.

A first-aid kit

You should have a first-aid kit for your dog. Commercially made kits are available but, in my opinion, these often do not contain the most important items that you will really need in an emergency.

My advice is to make up your own first-aid kit, guided by your vet or a veterinary nurse. Take it whenever you go away with your dog, and make sure that all members of your family know how to use it. Your first-aid kit should include the following:

1 Sheet of bubble-wrap
2 Cotton wool
3 Moist face-wipes
4 Adhesive bandages
5 Conforming bandages
6 Disposable gloves
7 Veterinary antiseptic
8 Muzzle (see page 98)
9 Impregnated gauze
10 5 ml and 10 ml syringes
11 Foil blanket
12 Washing-soda (sodium carbonate) crystals (see page 121)
13 Spare collar and lead
14 Salt (for bathing wounds)
15 Heat-generating pads
16 Length of cord for use as emergency muzzle (see page 99)
17 Sterile dressings
18 Thermometer
19 Curved, round-ended scissors
20 Long-handled, fine tweezers
21 Magnifying glass
22 Small torch and spare batteries
23 Pliers (or wire-cutters)
24 Pen-knife

Preventing accidents

By being a diligent and safety-conscious owner, you may be able to prevent your dog from being involved in some of the most common accident-and-emergency situations. Use your common sense, but remember in particular the following points:

• Ensure that your house and garden are escape-proof.
• When out and about near roads or other hazards, keep your dog on his lead.
• Be aware of potential hazards in your home and garden, such as trailing wires, chemicals, medicines, ponds, open garden sheds and rubbish bins.
• Do not leave your dog unsupervised with small toys or any other objects that he could destroy and swallow.
• Train your dog to respond immediately to your commands – especially to leave objects alone, to come back to you when called and to drop anything that he may be carrying in his mouth.
• Accustom your dog to regular health-checks from a young age (see pages 8–9), so that he is happy to have the most sensitive parts of his body examined.
• Never let your dog swim in water that you would not venture into yourself.
• When travelling with your dog in a car, make sure that he is properly restrained. He should either wear a proper car-safety harness that attaches to one of the rear seat belts (see page 29), or he should be behind a suitable dog-guard or in a proper car cage for dogs.

A ROAD ACCIDENT

1 Ask another person – if someone is available – to warn the approaching traffic of the accident.
2 Send someone to telephone a vet centre.
3 Approach your dog very quietly and slowly (see page 115).
4 If he has collapsed and appears to be unconscious, check whether or not he is breathing by watching his chest for movement. If you are in any doubt, pluck a small tuft of fur from his coat and hold it directly in front of his nostrils.
5 If your dog is not breathing, check that his airway is clear. Open his mouth and look right down to the back of his throat. Remove any obvious obstructions and pull his tongue forward.
6 If there is no obvious obstruction, extend your dog's neck by lifting up his chin and then, holding his mouth closed, give him mouth-to-nose artificial respiration. To do this, take a breath of fresh air and then gently breathe out into your dog's nostrils, at a rate of approximately 30 breaths per minute.
7 Check for a heartbeat or pulse (see opposite).
8 If you cannot feel either a heartbeat or pulse, begin chest compressions. If your dog is smaller than a West Highland white terrier, place one hand on either side of his chest, just behind his elbow, and squeeze your hands together to compress his chest. Do this at a rate of two compressions per second. If you have a larger dog, you will need to use a slightly different technique (see opposite, above). Every four compressions, give your dog artificial respiration for two breaths. Keep checking for a heartbeat or pulse, and only stop compressing the chest when you are able to feel a consistent pulse, or when veterinary assistance arrives.
9 If your dog is still conscious, apply an emergency muzzle (see page 99). However, DO NOT muzzle your dog if he is experiencing obvious difficulty in breathing, or if he has any injuries to his muzzle or jaw. Dogs with very flat faces cannot be muzzled. The best way to restrain a dog of this type is to wrap a twisted towel or an article of clothing around his neck for someone else to hold. Take care not to over-tighten the towel as

If your dog is injured, you must keep him warm. If you have your first-aid kit, wrap him in the foil blanket or bubble-wrap; otherwise, place a thick, warm coat over him.

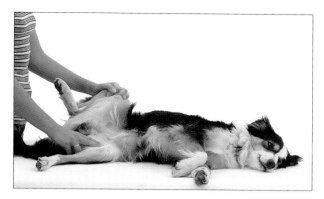

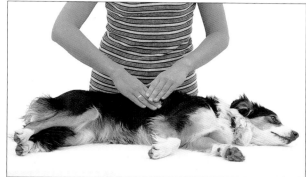

To check whether your dog's heart is beating, try to feel for his heartbeat by holding your fingers firmly against his chest on the left side, just behind his elbow; alternatively, you can try to feel for a pulse on your dog's inner thigh (as shown). As with other techniques described in this section, you should practise this procedure so that you will know how to locate your dog's pulse quickly in an emergency.

If you are sure that your dog's heart has stopped, you should begin chest compressions (DO NOT do this if he may have a chest injury). Apply intermittent pressure in a 'cough-like' manner to the chest wall, at a rate of two compressions per second. Position your hands as shown on a large dog; for a small dog see step 8, opposite. Every four compressions, give artificial respiration for two breaths (see step 6, opposite).

you do this, or you may cause your dog other problems, including breathing difficulties.

10 If your dog is bleeding, apply pressure to the source of any haemorrhage. If you have your first-aid kit, use a large pad of cotton wool bound firmly to the area with a conforming bandage. Otherwise, use a piece of clothing and apply pressure with your hands. If blood soaks through the dressing, do not remove it as you may disrupt any clots that have formed. Simply apply another dressing on top.

11 Cover any other open wounds to prevent them from becoming contaminated with dirt. If a skin

wound has a broken bone or bones protruding through it, apply a doughnut-shaped ring-pad dressing made from a bandage, scarf or any other suitable piece of material (see below).

12 If you think that your dog may have a broken leg and you have no choice but to move him, splint the broken leg first if at all possible. A tightly rolled-up newspaper, a piece of wood, a car-wheel brace or even a car-steering-wheel immobilizer will make a suitable temporary splint. Place the splint against the affected limb on the opposite side to any open wound, and bandage it firmly in place.

Making a ring-pad bandage

Use this type of bandage to protect a wound with a protruding bone or an impaled foreign body. A conforming bandage (see page 115) or a scarf will be suitable.

1 Wind the bandage around your hand three times, then take it off your hand and wind the rest of the bandage around the circle.

2 Tuck in the end of the bandage, and smooth out any wrinkles.

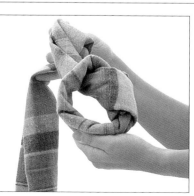

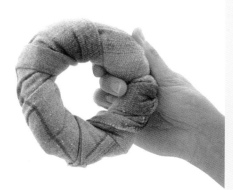

Moving an injured dog

To move an injured dog without causing further injury, use a stretcher if possible. The best type is a flat piece of wood or other rigid object such as a door or a gate. Lie this next to your dog, then slide him on to it by grasping handfuls of fur along his back. If no such object is available, make a sling from a sheet or rug.

If you are on your own, you may have to carry your dog. Place a forearm behind his hindlegs as if he is going to sit on your arm, and hold on to his knee joint on the side of his body that is furthest away from you. Put your free arm under his neck, across his chest, and then grasp his elbow on the side away from you.

No matter how you move your dog, your main aim should be to create as little movement in his body as possible, to avoid causing further injury and pain.

A SEVERE SKIN WOUND

1 If the wound contains one or more foreign bodies and is bleeding, try to remove any obvious foreign body that could be driven deeper into the wound by a pressure dressing, then apply a dressing of this type as quickly as possible (see step 10, page 117). Bright-red blood spurting from the wound is a sure sign that an artery has been severed: in this case, apply a pressure dressing immediately to the source of the spurt.
   • If the wound is not bleeding, leave any foreign body alone, or you may cause further damage and bleeding in trying to remove it. Instead, make a ring-pad dressing that is large enough to surround the entire wound (see page 117).
   • If a large foreign body – such as a piece of glass – is protruding a long way through the skin, carefully bandage around it.
2 If the wound does not appear to contain any foreign bodies, but is bleeding, apply a pressure dressing straight away (see step 10, page 117).
3 If the wound does not appear to contain any foreign bodies and is not bleeding, gently bathe it with an antiseptic solution and dry the area. Apply a protective dressing using impregnated gauze wrapped with plenty of cotton wool, compressed with a conforming bandage. If at any stage of the cleaning and washing procedure, the wound begins to bleed, stop and apply a pressure dressing as soon as possible (see step 10, page 117).
4 If you can move your dog and you think that it is safe to do so, take him to your vet centre as soon as possible. Otherwise, wait for your vet to arrive.

COLLAPSE

If your dog appears to be unconscious and is totally unaware of your presence, do the following:

1 Check whether he is breathing (see page 116).
2 If he is not breathing, check his throat for foreign bodies or swellings. If none is obvious, begin artificial respiration (see step 6, page 116).
3 Check for a heartbeat or pulse (see page 117). If you cannot detect a heartbeat or pulse, begin chest compressions (see pages 116–17).
4 Contact your vet centre as soon as possible.

If your dog is conscious, keep him calm, quiet and warm while you wait for help to arrive.

BREATHING DIFFICULTY OR CHOKING

1 Immediately check in your dog's mouth for any obvious foreign body. Do not poke about in his mouth without looking into it first, or you may push a foreign body back into his throat.

Playing 'fetch' games with sticks can be dangerous, as many dogs have accidentally impaled themselves in the throat when picking a stick up from the ground on the run.

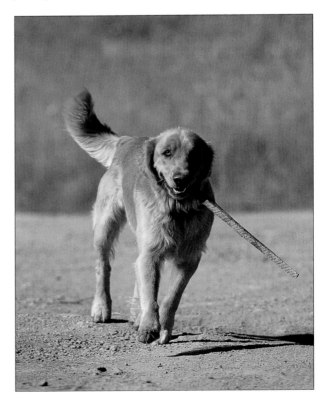

2 If there is a foreign body in your dog's mouth, try to remove it, but watch your fingers (you may need someone's help to keep your dog's mouth open). If the object is deep in his throat, leave it alone or you may push it further towards his airway.

3 Quickly lift up your dog's hindlegs, so that he is standing on his forelegs with his head down. Rest his hindlegs over your knee or the arm of a chair, and squeeze his chest five times, with a hand on either side of his rib cage, in sharp, 'cough-like', jerking movements. Only move your hands a little, in order to stimulate a sudden rush of air from his lungs: this should help to dislodge a foreign body that is stuck at the back of his throat. If you have a small dog or a puppy, use the first two fingers of each hand and be sensible about the amount of pressure that you apply.

4 As soon as your dog coughs out the foreign body, settle him on the floor and let him calm down in his own time. Do not stimulate him, and discourage him from moving.

5 Contact your vet centre to tell your vet what has happened. There is little point in doing so sooner, as this will waste precious time: your dog's best chance of survival rests with you.

LACK OF CO-ORDINATION/ 'DRUNKEN' BEHAVIOUR
(See also possible poisoning on page 120, strange behaviour on page 121 and heatstroke on page 123.)

1 Try to prevent your dog from moving about.
2 Restrict him to a darkened and quiet room. Stay with him, but do not stimulate him in any way.
3 Contact your vet centre.

A SEIZURE (CONVULSION OR 'FIT')
(See also page 79.)

1 If your dog is indoors, darken the room and keep the surrounding area quiet.
2 Contact your vet centre.
3 Stay with your dog, but do not touch him unless he is about to injure himself. In this case, move him carefully so as to stimulate him as little as possible.
4 Even if you think that he may be choking on his tongue or about to bite it, do not handle your dog's mouth: he may bite you by accident.
5 Your dog should stop fitting after a few minutes, but continue to observe him. Do not move him or encourage him to move by himself. If he does get up, do not try to stop him as your restraint may stimulate him to have another seizure.

AN UNPLANNED MATING

If you have an unspayed bitch and you think that she may have been involved in an unplanned mating, contact your vet centre immediately. If you can do so within 24 to 96 hours of the mating, your vet may be able to give her an injection to prevent an unwanted pregnancy.

---

6 If your dog continues to fit, or comes out of one fit and goes straight into another, keep observing him and wait for your vet to arrive.

SUDDEN, SEVERE VOMITING
(See also pages 28–9.)

1 Make sure that your dog does not attempt to eat or drink anything.
2 Contact your vet centre.
3 Each time your dog vomits, note down the time, and the consistency and quantity of the vomit that he produces (keep him inside on newspaper, so that you can see this). This information may help your vet to identify the cause of the problem and to devise appropriate treatment.

SUDDEN, SEVERE DIARRHOEA
(See also pages 30–1).

1 Make sure that your dog does not eat.
2 Contact your vet centre.
3 Each time your dog passes diarrhoea, note down the time, and the consistency and quantity of what he produces (you should keep him indoors on newspaper so that you can monitor him). Providing this information may help your vet to identify the cause of the problem and to treat it accordingly.

A HEAT BURN
1 Immediately cool the affected area as quickly as possible, by thoroughly soaking it with cold, running water for at least 10 minutes. While you are doing so, contact your vet centre.
2 Cover the affected area in cling film, then wrap up your dog to keep him warm. If you have a foil blanket or bubble-wrap, use this with blankets.

A CHEMICAL BURN
1 Muzzle your dog (see pages 98–9) to prevent him from licking his skin.
2 Wash the affected area of skin with copious amounts of running water (as above). While you are doing so, contact your vet centre.

INGESTION OF A POSSIBLE POISON

If you think that your dog may have ingested a poisonous substance, contact your vet centre as soon as you have carried out emergency care, as outlined below. Do not attempt to make your dog vomit (see opposite) unless there is a clear indication to do so – if in doubt, don't.

If possible, tell your vet the name of the substance that your dog has swallowed. If your vet is not familiar with the product, a veterinary nurse may be able to find out more information while you are on your way to your vet centre. Take the product packaging with you.

CORROSIVE ACIDS

Examples include the liquid from a car battery, or a chemical kettle descaler.

Administer a dilute solution of sodium bicarbonate (2.5 ml [half a teaspoonful] in 250 ml [8 fl oz] of water) by mouth to help to neutralize the corrosive chemical.

DO NOT attempt to make your dog vomit.

CORROSIVE ALKALIS

Examples include paint stripper, oven-cleaning chemicals and creosote.

Administer vinegar (diluted 50:50 with water) or orange juice to your dog by mouth to help to neutralize the corrosive chemical.

DO NOT attempt to make your dog vomit.

IRRITANTS

Examples include decaying meat, some plants (dumb cane, poinsettia, laburnum) and chemicals (lead, arsenic, mercury).

DO NOT attempt to make your dog vomit.

NARCOTICS

Examples include human barbiturates (dogs seem to like the taste of these), turpentine and paraffin.

If you see your dog eat a narcotic substance, try to make him vomit immediately (see opposite, above).

If you believe that your dog may have eaten a narcotic substance, but you did not see him do it and you do not know when he may have done so, DO NOT try to make him vomit: there is a chance that his swallow reflex may be affected, which could cause him to inhale his vomit.

Try to keep your dog awake by constantly stimulating him until veterinary help arrives.

CONVULSANTS

Examples include slug bait (metaldehyde), anti-freeze (ethylene glycol) and laurel leaves.

If you see your dog eat and swallow a convulsant substance, or you believe that he has done so, try to make him vomit immediately (see opposite, above).

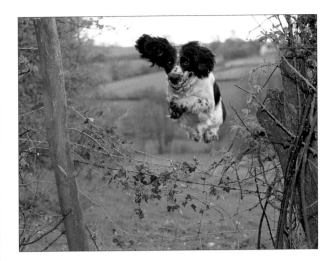

Given the athletic lifstyle that many dogs enjoy, it is hardly surprising that they receive bruises, cuts and scratches. In general, paws, legs and heads are especially prone to injury.

SEVERE LAMENESS
(See also pages 44–5.)
1 Immediately restrict your dog's movement.
2 If he cannot bear any weight on the affected leg, if it looks an unusual shape or if it is very swollen, contact your vet centre immediately.
3 Only move your dog if absolutely necessary: for instance, to get him to your car. If he cannot walk on three legs, you must carry him (see page 118).
4 If your dog will not keep the affected leg still, splint the leg (see page 117); if he can bear some weight on the leg, refer to pages 44–5.

APPARENT PARALYSIS
1 If your dog does not seem to be able to stand up, or can only raise his front end off the ground, contact your vet centre immediately.
2 Stay with your dog and keep him calm, quiet and warm. Do not attempt to move him.

A SUDDEN, SEVERE SKIN SWELLING
Your dog may develop a skin swelling for a number of reasons. Two accidental causes of swellings that may have serious results are insect stings and snake bites.

Due to a wasp/bee sting
1 If the sting is in your dog's mouth, nose or throat, seek veterinary attention for him immediately, as any swelling may block his airway.

2 If your dog has been stung by a bee, the sting may still be in his skin. If you can see the sting, carefully grasp it close to the skin, using a pair of tweezers, and remove it. As you do this, try not to squeeze or break the poison sac, as this could pump more of the bee's poison into your dog.

3 You can help to neutralize the effects of a bee sting by bathing the area with a solution made up of 10 ml (1 dessertspoonful) of bicarbonate of soda and 600 ml (1 pint) water. For a wasp sting, use vinegar diluted 50:50 with water. If these substances are not available, soap and water should relieve the pain.

4 Apply a cold compress, such as a cloth wetted with very cold water (packed with ice if possible), or a bag of frozen peas, to try to control the swelling.

Due to a snake bite

1 If you see your dog being bitten by a snake, or you think that he may have been bitten (especially by an adder in the UK), quickly carry him home, or to your car if you are out on a walk.

2 Keep him as still as possible. If he moves about, he may increase the speed with which the venom spreads from the bite wound to the rest of his body.

3 Contact your vet centre as soon as possible.

4 Gently wash the area of the bite wound with soap and water (this will help to relieve the pain).

5 Apply a cold compress, such as a cloth wetted with very cold water, or a bag of frozen peas, to try to control the swelling.

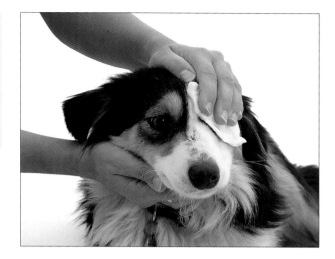

If your dog's eye is swollen or bleeding, gently cover it with a pad of cotton wool soaked in cold water. Keep the injured eye covered like this until your vet is able to examine it.

AN EYE INJURY

1 Prevent your dog from rubbing his eye as, by doing so, he is likely to cause further damage.

2 Look closely for any foreign body, such as a piece of stalk or grit, that may be trapped behind the upper or lower eyelid (use a magnifying glass if necessary). If you can see a foreign body, try to flush it out by pouring warm water gently over the eye, but, if this distresses your dog further, stop. Never try to remove a foreign body from your dog's eye, as you could cause further damage.

3 Contact your vet centre.

4 If the eye is swollen, apply a cold compress in the form of a cloth wetted with very cold water.

STRANGE BEHAVIOUR

(See also lack of co-ordination on page 119.)

1 Examine your dog to see if there is anything obvious that may be wrong with him physically.

2 Try to identify anything unusual in his environment that may be upsetting him.

3 Contact your vet centre for advice.

4 If your dog's behaviour is particularly strange, videotape it if possible, as he may not behave in the same way at your vet centre.

SUDDEN ABDOMINAL SWELLING

If your dog's abdomen suddenly appears swollen (see left), seek veterinary attention immediately.

COAT CONTAMINATION
(See also a chemical burn on page 119.)

First of all, muzzle your dog (see pages 98–9) to prevent him from licking his coat, as the offending substance may be poisonous or may burn his mouth.

Whatever the kind of contamination, check the underlying skin for burns and treat as necessary (see page 119). Contact your vet centre if the skin looks inflamed, if you cannot remove the contaminant, if you think that your dog may have ingested some of the substance, or if he is unwell in any other way.

Non-oily compounds
An example is a disinfectant solution.
1 Wash your dog's coat with plenty of water. (DO NOT use any form of detergent, as this may increase the speed with which any toxic chemical is absorbed through the skin.)

Liquid, oily compounds
Examples are engine oil and creosote.
1 Smear the affected area with a commercial hand-cleaning jelly, or with liquid-paraffin or cooking oil.
2 Wash the area with a detergent, such as washing-up liquid, and warm water. Rinse thoroughly, then repeat as many times as necessary. (DO NOT use petrol or any other inflammable liquid.)

Solid oily compounds
An example is tar.
1 If possible, carefully clip off the contaminated hair.
2 Alternatively, rub commercial hand-cleaning jelly, liquid-paraffin or cooking oil into the affected area and treat as for a liquid, oily compound (see above).

FOREIGN BODIES
A foreign body may be defined as any object in a place in which you would not normally expect to find it. As a result of their activities, some dogs are very prone to picking up all kinds of foreign bodies.

Gagging
1 If your dog cannot close his mouth, is drooling excessively or appears to be gagging, immediately take a look inside his mouth.
2 If you can see a foreign body, attempt to remove it using a pair of tweezers (avoid using your fingers if at all possible). If there seems to be a piece of bone or another object jammed between your dog's teeth across the roof of his mouth, only try to remove it if you have a helper to hold your dog's mouth open

and a suitable pair of tongs or pliers to try to grasp it. Push the object backwards to loosen it, before very carefully removing it from your dog's mouth.
3 If you are not able to remove the foreign body quickly and easily, or your dog becomes distressed, contact your vet centre immediately.

A foreign body in the nose
If you see a foreign body protruding from one of your dog's nostrils, do not attempt to remove it. The object may be longer than you think, and by trying to remove it you may inadvertently break it off inside his nose.

Violent head-shaking
If your dog is shaking his head violently, he may well have a foreign body in his ear. Do not poke anything into his ear hole. Contact your vet centre immediately.

A swallowed foreign body
(See also pages 34–5.)
1 Make sure that your dog does not eat or drink.
2 Contact your vet centre immediately.

A foreign body in the anus
1 Muzzle your dog, and ask an assistant to restrain him for you (see pages 98–100).
2 Examine the foreign body. If it looks sharp, leave it alone; if not, grasp it with tweezers and gently pull it. If there is any resistance at all, stop immediately.
3 Contact your vet centre.

BLEEDING FROM THE MOUTH
1 Examine your dog to locate the source of the blood.
2 If you identify a foreign body, only try to remove it if it is not stuck hard into the gums, tongue or cheeks. If you can see a foreign body but cannot remove it, or you cannot identify the cause of the bleeding, contact your vet centre immediately.
3 If the quantity of blood is small and there is no obvious cause, keep your dog calm and quiet. Monitor him for the next 10 minutes. If the bleeding does not stop, or worsens, contact your vet centre.

A BROKEN TOOTH

Although a dog who has a broken tooth (or teeth) may continue to eat as normal, do not imagine that this is not a painful problem: it is. If you notice that your dog has a broken tooth, you should contact your vet centre as soon as possible to arrange prompt treatment.

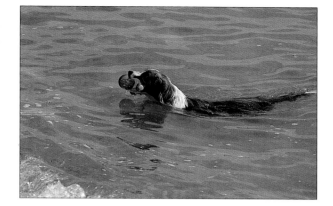

STRAINING TO PASS URINE

If your dog is straining but is not passing any urine at all, contact your vet centre immediately. If he is passing small amounts of urine frequently, try to obtain a sample in a clean container, as this will help your vet to diagnose the problem. Then contact your vet centre during normal hours.

STRAINING TO PASS FAECES

Contact your vet centre as soon as possible, and try to prevent your dog from continually straining by distracting him, as he may cause further problems.

HEATSTROKE

If your dog is suffering from heatstroke, he will be restless, very distressed and will pant excessively. As his condition worsens, he will start to drool and will become unsteady on his feet.

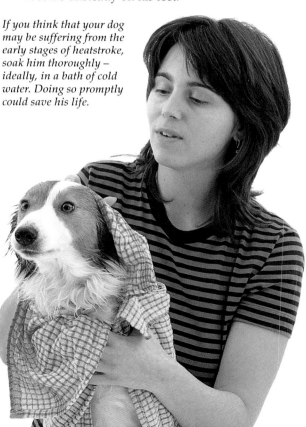

If you think that your dog may be suffering from the early stages of heatstroke, soak him thoroughly – ideally, in a bath of cold water. Doing so promptly could save his life.

Many dogs love to swim. If yours is one of them, train him to wait until you allow him to wade in. Do not let him swim in fast-moving or stagnant water, or where there is no easy exit.

1 If you suspect heatstroke, cool your dog down immediately using cold-water baths or by soaking him with running water.
2 Cover him with soaked blankets or towels, and continue to douse him with water.
3 Contact your vet centre immediately.

DROWNING

1 If you are able to rescue your dog, immediately turn him upside-down to drain the water from his lungs. If you can, hold him up and off the ground by his hindlegs; if he is heavy, rest his legs over a fence.
2 If your dog is not breathing, begin artificial respiration (see step 6, page 116). Between breaths, check for a heartbeat or pulse. If you cannot feel either, begin chest compressions (see pages 116–17).
3 Contact your vet centre as soon as possible. If you are on your own, call out to attract the attention of someone who will be able to help you.
4 If your dog begins to cough, splutter and breathe on his own, dry him off and keep him warm.

AN ELECTRIC SHOCK

1 Switch off the electricity.
2 If your dog is not breathing, begin artificial respiration (see step 6, page 116). Between breaths, check for a heartbeat or pulse. If you cannot feel either, begin chest compressions (see pages 116–17).
3 Contact your vet centre.
4 If your dog is still breathing, or you manage to resuscitate him, keep him calm, treat any burns (see page 119) and wrap him up to keep him warm.

The end of your dog's life

Your dog is one of the family, and you and all those who have shared his life will be devastated when he dies. Before coming to terms with your loss, you will inevitably ride an emotional roller-coaster that may take you through stages of shock and disbelief, sadness, anger, yearning and depression. In your mind you will re-live many of the events from your dog's life, including those immediately prior to his death.

When your dog has gone, you will miss him more than you could ever imagine possible. However, it is important – particularly for the sake of any children you may have – that you handle your dog's death so as to minimize the grief that you all feel and to maximize the fond memories.

EUTHANASIA

Your dog may die suddenly and unexpectedly as a result of an accident or an acute illness, or he may be fortunate enough to pass away quietly in his sleep as a happy old man. However, if he is terminally ill and suffering unnecessarily – at any age – you should be brave enough to do the right thing, and to agree to your vet putting your dog out of his misery by ending his life through euthanasia.

What is euthanasia?

Often inappropriately described as 'putting a dog to sleep', euthanasia is the painless and premature ending of a dog's life, to prevent him from continuing to suffer from the pain, discomfort and misery of terminal illness or untreatable injury. It can only be carried out by a vet, and normally involves injecting a lethal dose of an anaesthetic drug directly into the bloodstream through the cephalic vein on the foreleg. The dog will lose consciousness and die within just seconds of the injection being given; all he will feel is a slight scratch as the needle penetrates his skin.

Deciding on euthanasia

The decision to euthanase your dog is one that you should make together with all the members of your family and your vet. Before making a decision one way or the other about your dog's future, you should be fully aware of the seriousness of his condition and of each of the options that exists.

The following are the kinds of questions to which you should obtain clear and precise answers:
• What is wrong with my dog, and is he in pain?
• Will he recover?
• What could be done to help control his symptoms?
• What quality of life would this treatment give him?
• What kind of special nursing will he need?
Your dog's condition may be such that euthanasia is clearly the only option open, but most owners of terminally ill dogs are faced with a more difficult decision. Your vet will of course give you his or her recommendation as to which course of action is most appropriate, but the final decision must be yours.

Taking your time

Unless your dog's present condition dictates otherwise (for instance, if he is seriously injured in an accident), do not feel pressurized to make an immediate decision about his future. It is very important that you consider carefully everything that your vet has told you, and that you discuss all the options as a family.

For each option, think what your dog's quality of life will be. Will he be living, or simply existing? Try as hard as you can to ignore your own feelings: you must do what is right for your dog. Many owners later regret having kept their terminally ill dogs alive simply because they could not face saying goodbye. If you cannot reach a decision, ask dog-owning friends and relatives what they would do, as they will be able to

Older children should be involved in a decision on euthanasia. If they do not understand why and how your dog has died, and they do not have the chance to say goodbye, they will grieve all the more.

consider your dog's condition from a more detached perspective. Take the time that you need. If you do decide to euthanase your dog and you know that you have made the right decision, you will be less likely to compound your grief with feelings of guilt.

What happens next?

If you do decide that euthanasia is the right option, your vet or a veterinary nurse will help you to make the necessary arrangements. Your dog's euthanasia can be carried out either at your vet centre or at your own home: the decision should be yours. My own feeling is that – if at all possible – it is most appropriate for a dog to die at home, in familiar surroundings.

Who should be there?

Only you as a family can make that decision. Very rarely are there any complications in euthanasia, but you should be aware that, if your dog's circulation is very poor, it may be difficult for your vet to locate a vein in which to give the injection. Some owners prefer to leave the room while the procedure is carried out, but return afterwards to see their dogs at peace.

Saying goodbye

No matter where your dog is euthanased, or whether you will be present, all the family should try to say a final goodbye, as this will help you to cope with your sense of loss. When, where and how you do so is up to you. Some owners prefer to say goodbye to their dogs before they are euthanased; others find it easier and more appropriate to hold some kind of simple ceremony that is meaningful to them.

AFTER YOUR DOG'S DEATH

Whether your dog dies naturally or by euthanasia, you will have to decide what to do with his body. If you wish to bury him in your garden or in another special place, you should check first with your local environmental-health authority that you are allowed to do so. It may be possible where you live to bury your dog in a special pet cemetery.

Cremation

Most owners choose to have their dogs cremated: your vet centre should be able to arrange this for you. If you wish, your dog's ashes can then be returned for burial.

One old man who went fishing with his dog every day could never stop the dog from jumping overboard on the way back and swimming the last few hundred metres back to the jetty. When his dog died, the man

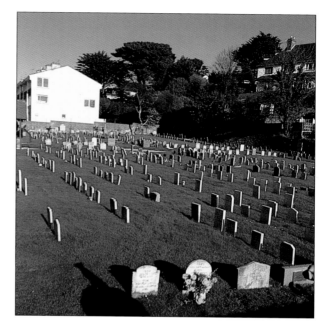

Pet cemeteries are now quite commonplace in some countries. Their existence is proof enough that dogs hold a very special place in their owners' hearts, even long after they have died.

had his dog cremated and took his ashes out with him on his next fishing trip. When he reached the place where his dog used to leap into the water, he emptied the ashes over the side, and, by saying farewell in this way, took a vital step in coping with his grief.

Even if you decide not to have your dog's ashes returned, you and your family may like to hold some kind of ceremony to celebrate your dog's life and to acknowledge his death. Burying his collar and lead and planting a special shrub in your garden may make you feel better. Encourage your children to cry openly if they wish, and lead by example.

BEREAVEMENT COUNSELLORS

If you find that you are not coping very well with your dog's death, and that your sadness is affecting other areas of your life, you must talk to someone who understands what you are going through. Contact your vet centre, and speak to your vet or to a veterinary nurse whom you know well. He or she may decide to put you in touch with a bereavement counsellor, who will help you to come to terms with your loss.

Index

ACKNOWLEDGEMENTS

The publishing of any book is a team effort, and I would like to express my sincere thanks to the many organizations and individuals – both human and canine – that have played a part in creating *Dog Doctor*.

I am particularly indebted to the following friends and colleagues for their general advice and guidance, and for their specific contributions:

David Ashworth BVetMed MRCVS
Serena Brownlie Phd BVMS CertSAC MRCVS
Steve Butterworth MA VetMB CertVR DSAO MRCVS
Elspeth Down BVetMed MRCVS
John Down BVetMed MRCVS
Hugh Duffin BVetMed MRCVS
Jonathan Elliot NA VetMB Phd CertSAC MRCVS
Gary England BVetMed Phd DVR CertVA MRCVS
Maxine Field VN
Peter Holt BVMS Phd CBiol DipECVS MIBiol FRCVS
Janet & Craig Irvine-Smith BVSc (Pret) MRCVS and all the staff of the Stonehenge Veterinary Hospital
Morag Kerr BVMS BSc Phd MRCVS
Richard Laven BVetMed MRCVS
Andrew Lawley BSc BVetMed MRCVS
Ben Linnell BVetMed MRCVS
Chris Little BVMA Phd Cert SAC MRCVS
Joanna Morris BSc BVetMed MRCVS
Sue Oxley VN
Simon Petersen-Jones DVetMed DVOphthal MRCVS
John Robinson BDS (Lond)
Gairn Ross BVMS MRCVS and the 180 veterinary surgeons of the People's Dispensary for Sick Animals (PDSA)
David Scarff BVetMed CertSAD MRCVS
Jim Simpson SDA BVMS Mphil MRCVS
David Watson BVetMed MRCVS
David Williams MA VetMB CertVOphthal MRCVS
The Publishing Team Sam, Viv, Jane, Alyson, Claire and Nina.

PUBLISHER'S ACKNOWLEDGEMENTS

Mitchell Beazley would like to thank the following organizations and people for their help with photography, illustrations and modelling:

Mr A. Glue at Milbrooke Animal Centre (RSPCA), Chobham; Craig & Janet Irvine-Smith, Howard Taylor, Sue Holden, Liz McGauley and Anne Walton at Stonehenge Veterinary Hospital; Graham & Lesley Howlett & Ben (our star dog model!); Vicky Gray; Alison, Mike & Grace Molan; Sue Oxley; Shirley Arthur; Vera Lopez; Sarah Pollock, Nicola O'Connell; Tim Ridley; Rosie Hyde and Jane Burton.

PICTURE CREDITS

Animal Health Trust 52
University of Bristol/Department of Companion Animals/Dr Frances Barr 92 below
University of Bristol/Dept of Clinical Veterinary Science/Dr. John Innes 47 above left, 47 above right
University of Bristol/Dept. of Clinical Veterinary Science/Dr Paul Wotton 39 below left, 39 above left, 40 above right, 40 above left
University of Cambridge/The Queen's Veterinary School Hospital/Mr M Bostock 75
University of Edinburgh Dept of Veterinary Clinical Studies/Dr.A H M van den Broek 60
Jane Burton 1, 123 top
Sylvia Cordaiy/Paul Kaye 50
Celia Cox 18, 22
Gill Harris 42 above right, 94 top
Journal of Small Animal Practice/D.N. Carlotti 20 top / R.E.W. Halliwell 63
Leo Animal Health 62 below left
Oxford Scientific Films/Animals Animals 13 below/Carol L.Geake 33, 82/Daniel J Cox 118/London Scientific Films 32 below left/Okapia/J.L.Klein & M.L. Hubert 35 below/ David Tipling 120/Charles Tyler 125
Reed International Books Ltd/Jane Burton 2, 42 below left, 44, 46, 58 below left, 66 below right, 66 below left, 77 81 below, 98, 99 top left, top centre, top right, 100 below right, below left, 101 below right, below centre, below left, 102 top right, top left, below, 103 top left, top right, below, 104 below right, below left, 105, 106, 107 below, top left, top right, 109 below left, below right, top, 111 top, below, 115, 116, 117 below left, below right, top right, top left, 121, 123 below, 124 /Nick Goodall 58 below right/Rosie Hyde/Stonehenge Veterinary Hospital 21, 24 below, 31 top left, top right, 36, 45, 49 above left, above right, 55, 61, 65, 81 top, 83, 85, 89, 90, 91 below, top, 92 top left, top right, 93 below, top, 94 below, 95, 96, 97 below, top, 100 top, 108, 112, 113 top, below/Ray Moller 68, 69/Tim Ridley 3, 6, 7, 9 main pic, 9 insets top left, top right, top centre, below right, below left, 20 below, 64, 86, 87/Herb Schmitz 25, 29, 59, 99 below, 110 below, top
Jacket photography/Tim Ridley all except back right/ Rosie Hyde back right
Illustrations/Stefan Chabluk 70, 88/Liz Gray 27, 32, 33, 36, 39, 41, 47, 53, 59, 65, 72, 73, 80
John Robinson BDS (Lond) 24 top, 26, 27
Stonehenge Veterinary Hospital 51 top left, 51 top right
The Royal Veterinary College/Professor P. Bedford 13 top, 15, 16, 17
Yew Tree Veterinary Centre 35 top
You & Your Vet/Dr. R. Harvey 56, 62 top right
ZEFA Picture Library 14